MARIO LOPEZ'S
KNOCKOUT FITNESS

MARIO LOPEZ

with

Jeff O'Connell

RODALE

Rodale books may be purchased for business or promotional use or for special sales. For information, please write to:
Special Markets Department, Rodale Inc., 733 Third Avenue, New York, NY 10017

Printed in the United States of America
Rodale Inc. makes every effort to use acid-free ∞, recycled paper ♻.

Book design by Chris Rhoads

Cover and interior photography © Joan Allen

Library of Congress Cataloging-in-Publication Data is on file with the publisher
ISBN-13 978-1-59486-884-9
ISBN-10 1-59486-884-0

Distributed to the trade by Macmillan
2 4 6 8 10 9 7 5 3 1 hardcover

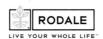

LIVE YOUR WHOLE LIFE™

We inspire and enable people to improve their lives and the world around them

For more of our products visit **rodalestore.com** or call 800-848-4735

Contents

Foreword
By **Oscar de la Hoya**

Mario Lopez is so full of energy that hanging out with him is as exhausting as surviving one of my title fights. Somehow, this guy is able to go full throttle 24/7 and still have something left in the tank, which never ceases to amaze me. I know professional fighters who can't match his stamina, perseverance, and determination. I've always wondered what his secret was, and now I know. You're holding it in your hands: *Mario Lopez's Knockout Fitness.*

Mario Lopez has the heart of champion, and boxing flows through his veins. He came out of the womb swinging and was throwing combinations in his crib. Yet this book is about so much more than boxing; in fact, that's only a small component of this fitness book. Above all, this is a serious workout program. I'd have to push it hard, but I could prepare for a title fight using the principles underlying *Knockout Fitness*: interval cardiovascular training and superset-based weight training. He and the remarkable team of experts he has assembled for this book somehow manage to tackle all of the body's energy systems simultaneously, sending your progress into warp drive.

What's unique and even extraordinary about Mario's approach to shaping up is that while it would work well for me and other boxers, it can work wonders for you too. Mario accommodates every preexisting fitness level. That's why it can work for everyone: men and women, young and old, the out of shape and the in shape, novice and advanced. What exactly do I mean by *work*? The program will make men look good—look like Mario—with lean cords of muscle, washboard abs, and body fat that's scarce and hard to find. The way boxers look before they step into the ring. It will make women look even better, with shape, tone, and definition to burn. Lean, sexy, and fit.

But Mario's program is about more than showing off a hot body. Your body is a tool, and this workout program is designed to make it work like a well-oiled machine, not a rusty farm implement. Sure, it will tighten your waist, but it will also boost your energy. Yes, it will build muscle, but it will also heighten your flexibility. You'll also become more explosive and more powerful, terms you'll understand in a fitness context once you have finished this book. Many personal trainers out there don't know as much about fitness as you'll know once you set down this book.

Knockout Fitness will work fast, too. If you're like me, progress that occurs at a glacial pace isn't progress at all because life passes you by in the meantime. What's more, it's fun. You'll love how Mario incorporates sports aside from boxing into his workout program. He's versatile as an entertainer, and his workouts are versatile too. There's never a dull moment when you're shaping up with my friend.

Mario is similar to boxers in that he takes a strategic approach to any endeavor. He's very discriminating when it comes to working out. He'll try anything once, but anything that doesn't work for him, he'll junk just as fast. I like his emphasis on whole-body training, because that's similar to how I train. His well-rounded workouts will produce a well-rounded body. With him, having shapely muscles or even a great looking physique isn't enough. You must be able to put it into action. His punches in the ring aren't spring-loaded because he has massive arms—although his arms are muscular—but because of his workouts.

Maybe it's the boxer in me, but one thing I admire about Mario is his ability to go the distance. Not all child actors were doomed to self-destruction ready-made for E! reenactment. This is a guy who started out on *Saved by the Bell*—a title any boxer has to love—and made that the foundation of a stellar career, something few child stars were able to do. Along with work ethic, what separated Mario from other child actors was his willingness to endure some short-term pain and sacrifice for long-term gain. That's the one thing he can't really teach, not even in this book: his tenacity and crazy intensity. Yet that drive and passion is unmistakable throughout *Knockout Fitness*.

Mario has faced a problem throughout his career that I can identify with: Sometimes it's hard for him to be taken seriously in the pursuit of his craft because of his looks. But he's a smart guy. Mario is well aware that if you want to look as good as he does into your 30s and beyond—even as career and family demands multiply—you need to be as economical as possible in the gym. That's how he came to develop his (relatively) short yet demanding sessions. His weight workouts are based around big moves that work many muscles at once. As for cardio, he came to favor interval training because that's what works best for decreasing body fat. When that bell sounds in boxing, there's no room for hesitation and self-doubt. When I watch Mario train, I see that see kind of spoon-bending focus on display.

Who is this book for?

If you hate working out, this is the program for you. With this book, you'll no longer be intimidated about hitting the gym. Take it one step at a time, and soon you'll be looking forward to the gym, not dreading it. This feeling will only intensify once you look in the mirror and see the changes wrought by Mario's program.

If you're lukewarm about working out, this is the program for you. Maybe you're one of those people who will train for a while, then stops for a while, and then picks it up again, without ever achieving anything approaching a true body transformation. You're going to stick with it this time because you'll finally make real progress.

If you love working out, this is the program for you. Even hardcore fitness people will be delighted by the new exercises, innovative programs, and delicious meal plans included in this book. You'll find instructions throughout if you're experienced and wanting to ramp it up a little faster than the average person will. Go for it!

Books are amazing things. They take a lifetime's worth of experience and knowledge and distill them into one volume that we can all carry with us wherever we go. Mario has compiled a resume full of amazing feats, but to me, this book you're holding in your hands right now stands as his most remarkable achievement to date. One thing that impressed me when I read Mario's manuscript is that he takes the science of exercise physiology and simplifies it so that everything is easy to understand it. I think that comes from his experience hosting. He never loses sight of his audience and need to connect with it at all times.

So step into the fitness ring with Mario and dedicate yourself to achieving the best shape of your life over the next six weeks. Your life will never be the same again.

Preface

My name is Mario Lopez, and I'm here to help you achieve the best shape of your life in as short a time as possible; and then stay fit for a really, really long time—like the rest of your life, which will last much longer as a result of the workouts you're about to follow.

That's a big promise, and promises certainly aren't in short supply these days where working out is concerned. After all, in today's world, slimming down has become big business. Whether we're watching TV, reading a magazine, or surfing the Internet, information hits us from every direction, 24/7, telling us what it takes to burn belly fat and build muscle—which is what men and women mean when they say, "I don't want to bulk up; I just want to get *toned*." You've heard that before, right—like a million times or so?

No, promises aren't in short supply. Results sure are, though. While the quantity of information would fill volumes, the quality of information leaves much to be desired. Which helps explain why so many people remain overweight and out of shape, with no idea how to really regain control of their body or their life. In fact, much of this workout information is nonsense, quite frankly. Fitness doesn't come from a fad workout, the protein bar of the month, or some magic powder (although nearly any workout sure beats the heck out of doing nothing, protein bars are useful, and well-designed supplements have their place in a smart diet). But the marketplace eats it up because everyone's looking for a shortcut these days. No one wants to put in the hard work. But there's no substitute for that.

If a shortcut is what you're after, you've come the wrong place. In fact, the single best piece of advice I can give you comes—Ta-da!—right now, in the fourth paragraph of the preface: There are no shortcuts to shaping up! But the second best piece of advice I can offer makes that first revelation easier to swallow: It doesn't matter that no shortcuts exist. That's what's so great about fitness. Pretenders fall by the wayside. You can't buy, cheat, or pray your way out of a gut or flabby chicken arms. You must put in the work. What's more, a shortcut would rob you what really matters: the journey.

You might ask why you should listen to the guy from *Saved by the Bell, Dancing with the Stars,* and *Extra!* when it seems like a million personal trainers and experts are putting forth workout programs and diets: some legit, some not so legit, and some ridiculous, in all honesty. I often rank high on those listings you see in supermarkets and on TV—you know, guys with the best bodies in Hollywood—but that's not why you should listen to me, and it's not the reason I chose to write this book. My look is merely a by-product of what I know and what I do. I don't work out to show off my abs at the beach, although I can't help it, either, if paparazzi use a zoom lens to shoot me with my shirt off on vacation. What can you do, right?

You should listen to me because the training and nutrition system you're about to follow is based on the most cutting-edge science available, and it works equally well for men and women, every single time, without fail. You should listen to me because while traveling along the path leading to this point, I've already made all the mistakes that I want you to avoid, starting with the summer before my senior year in high school, when I first picked up a weight. Working out the same muscle group over and over and over? Been there, done it. Not realizing how important sleep is? Affirmative. Eating the wrong things, and a lot of them, because I love food? Guilty as charged. Pushing it too far, listening to my ego instead of my body? Roger that. Throwing the weights around with no observance of correct form? Yep—in high school, especially, I really didn't know what I was doing. I didn't educate myself at all, at least not about working out.

Yet those long processes of trial and error, experimentation and discovery—and it's really the only way to learn—allowed me to figure out the hard way exactly what *does* work, and to know *why* it works. This book is my opportunity to share that knowledge with you, so that you can achieve the results I have, only more quickly. I welcome that opportunity.

This book is for everyone: men and women, young and old, fit and fat. Even if you're not overweight by any objective yardstick, you're not necessarily in tip-top shape. "Decent shape" and "well conditioned" are two different things. Take it from me: When I haven't been to the boxing gym consistently, I can tell that I don't have my wind and am not necessarily in peak condition. At other times, you think you're good shape, and then you do something different—in my case, being one of the contestants on the aforementioned *Dancing with the Stars*, for example. Suddenly, you feel muscles you've never felt before, or that you didn't even know existed. It quickly dawns on you that you're not really in as good a shape as you thought you were. It's a major wake-up call.

In other words, there's in shape, and then there's *in shape*.

This book's cover should probably displayed a red sticker: WARNING: THE AUTHOR OF THIS BOOK DOESN'T DO ANYTHING HALFWAY. IT'S ALL THE WAY OR NOTHING. Ever since I was a kid, I've put my heart and soul into every pursuit. I'm a driven guy by nature, and I'll be the first to admit it. Even if I have a day off, and I'm not feeling great, and I've been working on set all day . . . I've still got to do something physical, even if it's just going home to work the treadmill or smack around a punching bag. Call it an inner drive, or determination, or passion—call it whatever you want. But I simply cannot rest. Life's short. When I work hard, I work hard. When I party, I party hard. When I train, I train hard. My workouts are intense, and I love them for that very reason.

Yet working out does as much for my psyche as it does for my physique. I find it to be very therapeutic. I don't feel like I've ever really woken up unless I sweat. If I go more than two days without breaking a sweat or doing something physical, I'll start getting grumpy! I'm already a hyper guy, but powering through a workout gives me even more energy, which explains why I've been able to accomplish so much in 35 years. I raise the bar in the gym so I can go out and raise the bar in life. Training also helps me stare down stress. It bolsters my confidence in every other aspect of life. I just feel better all the way around when I'm working out consistently.

Now, I've taken those elements that work the best and merged them to create a program you can follow year-round, for the rest of your life. Best of all, my workouts, and the way I combine them, are fun. You're about to have a blast, trust me.

As we proceed through the book, I'll explain, in plainspoken, easy-to-understand language, exactly why I'm having you do the things you're doing. You deserve that if you're going to invest the time to work out, and change eating habits that may have been ingrained over the course of a lifetime. You need to be completely confident that what you're doing will produce the desired results. To not lift a finger is on you, but to do everything you're supposed to do, and have it not work, is in some ways even more dispiriting, because you *should* have shaped up! Heck, you made the effort. You paid the price. No money back guarantee can repay you for wasted time and postponed dreams.

In reality, while many people know they *should* work out, few people have a clue as to *how* they should work out. Before you head off to the gym, you need a plan like the one you hold in your hands now. If you walk in and arbitrarily do a little bit of this, a little bit of that, dabbling here, dabbling there, you won't accomplish anything of note. I'm a logical thinker by nature, so my attitude is, if you want something, first of all, you have to be realistic in laying out what it actually will take to achieve that goal. Think about homebuilders. Do they start hammering boards together and slapping together rooms? Of course not! They rely on blueprints to organize a collective effort into a finished product that not only looks great but also *works*. Building your body is similar to building a house. Start with a well-designed plan, and if you go in and execute, results will follow.

Part of making workouts fun is getting out of the gym once in a while. That way, when you do hit the gym doors, you'll want to be there, rather than feeling like a prisoner trapped forever in an iron dungeon. In this program, you'll find yourself running outside, hitting the beach, swimming, dancing, playing basketball, riding your bike—activities you normally associate with play, not work. (If you've never done these things before, don't worry, because I'm going to take you through them step by step.) But when the program sends you outside, you're being sent there for a reason. A lot of elements in this program are fun. Nothing in this program is random or unintentional.

Mixing the weights and cardio with sports activities not only makes the program fun—it also helps make you fit and toned in unique and unexpected ways. You can be the strongest man or woman in the gym, but if you tried to hold the rings like gymnasts do, your gym strength might be completely overmatched. The reverse might apply as well: The gymnast probably wouldn't be able to hoist up 180 pounds on the bench. It's a matter of what you're accustomed to—which explains why my program never lets you stagnate. Grow accustomed to a workout, and you stop growing. We'll have none of that here.

I love doing hill sprints, for example, and you'll be doing them, too. Fresh air and sunshine? You bet. That's one reason why hill work is so great. But a fascinating recent study in the *Journal of Strength and Conditioning Research* revealed that sprinting does more than just burn calories while your legs churn—it also increases your resting metabolic rate. Translation: You're not only burning more calories during the run itself than light jogging would allow, but that you're *still* burning extra calories long after the workout ends. Pumping gas on the way home from the gym? More calories burned. Shopping in the supermarket two hours later? Ditto. Watching TV that evening? You get the picture. By having you not just sprint, but sprint uphill, I'm sending your resting metabolism into overdrive. Soon enough, your body fat will melt like butter.

Is shaping up a matter of spending two hours a day in the gym, grunting through 100 sets or wearing out the treadmill, then crawling back to you car in the parking lot? Is it whiling away hours on a piece of cardio equipment like a gerbil works a spinning metal cylinder? Not even. Both of those approaches are doomed because they are a) extreme and b) as lopsided as that creaky roller. Gym goers these days usually choose one of two activities: cardiovascular exercise or resistance training—what we normally think of as lifting weights. I combine them. One minute I'll lift dumbbells, then I'll jump rope, then I'll work the heavy bag, then I'll do moves that wouldn't look out of place in a dance studio. What aggravates me more than anything is when I hear somebody say, "Well, I've got a secret exercise." There is no secret exercise. Power lifting, standard bodybuilding workouts, circuit training, heavy squats, cardio-sculpt classes—they all have their place, and I've done all of them, which is how I've come to know what works.

Before we proceed, let me offer a quick word to those of you, especially the ladies, who worry about bulking up on this program. Don't be afraid to lift weights, because you've got a long, long way to go before you need to worry about looking like a He-Man, or putting on too much muscle. Muscle is your means of burning fat. If you train to build, you'll start to lose weight, and then you'll start to trim. At the end of this program, you're going to be many things—lean, limber, and athletic, for starters—but muscle-bound isn't one of them.

When I train, I enter the gym, establish a rhythm, and accomplish what I need to accomplish, all in an hour or less. Then I go home. That's it. But that hour has to be used to its fullest, which requires focus. I don't take long breaks in between sets. I'm not one of those people who walk around the gym training only my jaws, chatting; and my neck, checking myself out in the mirror. (You know who you are, too!) When I'm there, I'm there for one reason and one reason only: to train hard. If a lot of the people I see at the gym spent as much time working out as they do socializing, they probably would look pretty great by now.

Do you have two hours a day to work out? I sure as heck don't. There are only 24 hours in a day, and some of those are for things like work and sleep. All I'm asking is that you take the time to take care of your body, and the return on that investment will be prodigious. You'll be amazed at how much more effective and productive you'll be during the other 23 hours, too.

(Yes, working out and eating right will improve your sleep. I'll explain why in Chapter 2, in the list 6 Reasons You Need 8 Hours of Sleep. In fact, skip ahead now if you want to check it out. Really, that's how I want you to read this book: dip in and out, double back, pick and choose, and skip around at will. This isn't a novel; it's a guidebook. Anyway, books aren't like diamonds—the paper and ink hold virtually no intrinsic value. So treat my workout book accordingly. In fact, six weeks from now, I hope this particular copy—the one you're holding in your hands right now—will be coffee-stained, dog-eared, and Post-It noted, the spine cracked and ink smudges from your thumbprints scattered throughout the pages. You know why? Because that will mean you're actually using it. In fact, if you ever hand this book to me at a signing, I want to see that you've beaten the heck out of it.)

You need to apply yourself fully to this endeavor, to channel your mental and physical energy into making fitness a priority. Don't let distractions take you away from the task at hand. It's not only about training, but also about preparing your food; eating what you should, and avoiding, or at least limiting, what you shouldn't; and getting sufficient rest. Tend to all that other stuff, and you'll achieve maximum results from your training.

Working out is about seeing how far you can go, about finding out what kind of stuff you're made of. What kind of character do you have? Are you going to buckle, or are you going to make it? That's what it's all about, whether you're a soldier trying to make it through Ranger School or a grandmother trying to run her first marathon. You have to take your body to the gym and sweat—that's the only way you're going to find out if you have what it takes.

By the way, that act of sweating itself will make you more attractive to the opposite sex. Researchers at the University of California, Berkeley, did a crazy experiment, in which they found that women become more turned on by viewing an erotic video after having smelled some of the body chemicals contained in male sweat. Who knew, right? In fact, female arousal rose threefold! And here you thought it was just because you looked so much better and were so much more confident. The same works in reverse, too: Nothing turns a guy on more than a woman shaping up in the gym.

Consider just one more great reason, among many, to bust a workout.

It's not only a matter of how you look, or how others perceive you; it's a matter of how you feel. In fact, as you shape up, I would argue that the changes occurring on the inside are even more important than the external transformation, as dramatic as that will be if you follow my workout program to the T. Those are two sides of one coin, of course. When you look better, the feedback you receive from those around you will make you feel better on the inside (not to mention the feedback you'll receive when you look in the mirror). The journey you embarked upon by buying this book is healthy for your body, mind, and soul alike. Stick with it, and next thing you know, if you're having a bad day, your troubles will just melt away along with your belly flab.

Hard work pays off. Your results are going to be over and above what your average Joe or Jane accomplishes in his or her workouts. In order for your body to fulfill its potential, you have to continually climb mountains. (I'm speaking metaphorically, but if you want to climb mountains for real, these workouts will hold you in good stead for that as well. In fact, that sounds like fun. I might try that myself.) You can never be happy with the workout you did yesterday. You need to be happy with the workout you're having today, and the one after that. That way, you're always moving forward.

Finally, aim high in your fitness goals, but don't adopt the all-or-nothing mentality that so many people have. Whether it's working out or dieting, small changes last, and big ones don't. If your schedule is crunched and you can only make it to the gym twice in a given week, that's better than once—and perhaps as good as three times, believe or not. A team of Canadian researchers recently did a study in which they divided subjects into those who did a workout spread over two days, and those who spread the same workout over three days. Lo and behold, those training two days progressed at a rate similar to those training an extra day.

Another team of exercise scientists, this time at the University of Kansas, found that beginner's can double their strength with only three 15-minute workouts a week. What's more, *96 percent* of these beginners were still training consistently six months later, a remarkable testament to the benefits of a slow-and-steady approach. Rome wasn't built in a day, and your body won't be either.

Always, always, always bear in mind the following dictum: When it comes to exercise, something trumps nothing every time, hands down. If I accomplish one thing in writing this book, it will be to drum that mantra into your head. That's why I've scattered 10-minute workouts throughout these pages. I developed them for those times when I had only a small window before a gig or call time, and they can work wonders for anyone on the go, including you. No excuses. Everyone can find ten minutes.

Here's the flipside to what I said about building according to a blueprint: You can have all the meal plans and workouts in the world scattered at your feet, but without dedication and motivation, they're worthless. You're just standing in a trash heap. As with anything else worth doing, dedication and motivation must be built over time. You can't just snap your fingers and change lifelong tendencies—that's why New Year's resolutions seldom last more than a few weeks or even days. Take the slow, steady route, and you'll reach your destination.

Moderation is a key to success; perfectionism is a prescription for failure, because none of us is perfectly disciplined all the time. I have setbacks and injuries, and so will you. Don't expect to enjoy smooth sailing all the time. The challenges you face won't all be internally generated, either. Obstacles stand in our way in life, and working around them is absolutely essential. Often, that's the crucial difference between those who are successful and those who lose their way.

Make the most of a situation, even if it's not ideal. Make your setbacks temporary by returning quickly to the gym, and you'll sustain momentum. And as you improve physically and mentally, the setbacks will become fewer and farther between. It's a virtuous cycle, not the vicious one that kicks in when you're out of shape to begin with, and the situation worsens by the day. Your biggest limitations spring from your mind.

For me, after nearly 20 years of dedicated training, I have adopted the words in this book as my lifestyle. I live this way 24/7. There's no turning back now. This isn't a burden I carry. I *can't wait* to work out each day. (I'm a boxer too, so just try keeping my out!) I look forward to eating a clean, nutritious meal instead of junk food. I'm a strong-willed person, but it depends on your motivation as well, on how badly you want it. It's nice to say, "I want to be a millionaire," or, "I want a body like a swimwear model's." Sure, who wouldn't? But then you have to ask, *If this is what it's going to take to get there, realistically, am I prepared to do that*? Other people don't do that; they're like, *Yeah, sure, I'd like to do that*. But do you realize what kind of commitment and time and sacrifice it will take?

When all is said and done, if you end up looking like me, good for you. Heck, look *better* than me. Please, be the person who knocks me off those best bodies lists. But don't obsess over a stomach so chiseled that you hear the wind whistling through the grooves separating your six-pack, or the proverbial buns of steel. Who wants buns of steel anyway?

So join me in this undertaking. If you stick with it, the journey will change your life like it has changed mine. You have my word on that.

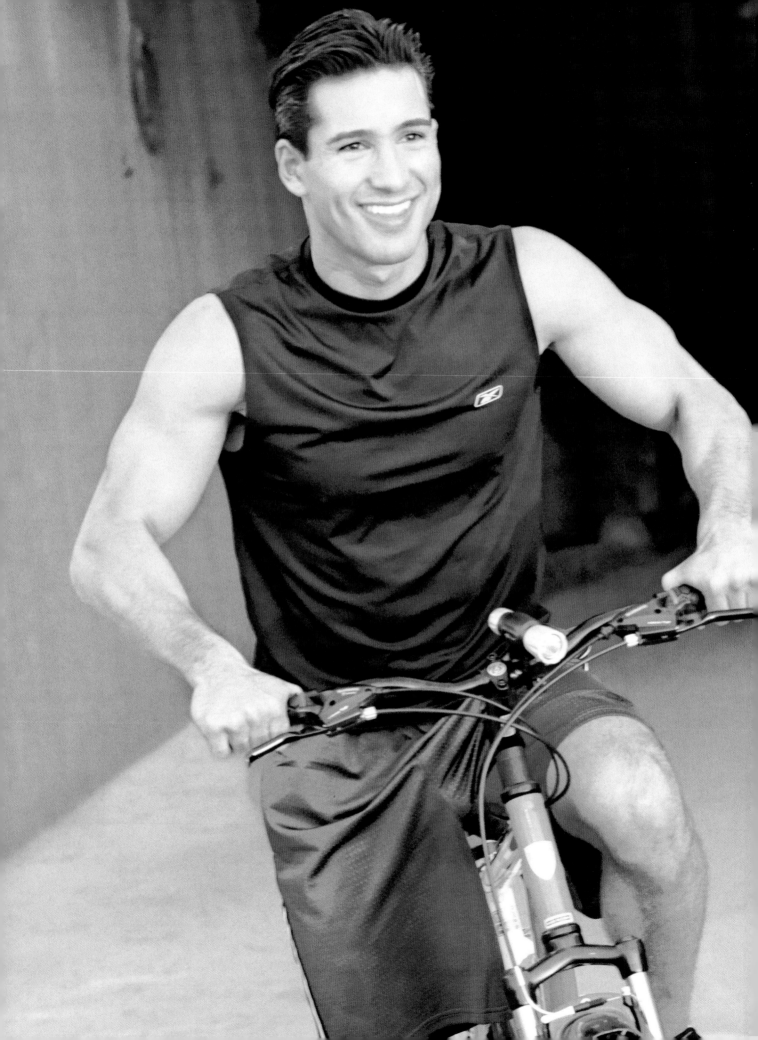

1

Form Meets Function

Check this out: I've been training now for going on two decades! So it shouldn't come as a surprise that my daily workouts, while a heck of a lot of fun, are fairly advanced and quite demanding. For many of you, those workouts would be impossible to ace right off the bat, and perhaps even unsafe, given their degree of difficulty. What we need to do is build you up to my level in a way that maximizes effectiveness, ensures safety—and guarantees that you have a blast in the process. Because if you're not having fun, you'll never stick with it. That's Mario's Rule of Fitness.

For those of you with at least some training experience, the Mario Lopez Knockout Fitness program lasts six weeks, divided among three two-week phases. However, complete beginners who will be entering a gym for the first time, or for the first time in a long while, will spend twice as long—four weeks—in each of the three phases, for 12 weeks total.

How do you determine your current fitness level? It can be tricky. Perhaps you *think* you're only a beginner, because you've only dabbled in the gym, when in fact you're actually an intermediate, perhaps because you're naturally a great athlete. The reverse can apply as well: You might not be as far along as you think.

I'm going to have you determine your "training age," which in turn will determine whether you spend two or four weeks in each phase. If you've been training for at least a year, you should be in relatively good shape—fit and strong enough to spend only two weeks in each phase. If you've been training for less than a year, follow the beginner sequence: four-by-four-by-four. The intermediate and advanced people will be doing the same phases as you beginners. They'll just be moving in and out of them much more quickly.

Don't become too hung up on the differences among beginning, intermediate, and advanced fitness people. Watch a show like *Dancing with the Stars*, and you'll see how quickly people can adapt to physical challenges—especially when they're having fun doing it! Think of it another way: There's no difference in Kobe Bryant shooting a free throw and Mario Lopez shooting a free throw. The difference comes in the level of commitment, focus, and dedication to performing it repetitiously over time. The difference between beginner and advanced is simply the amount of experience you have, say, doing a bench press or running on the treadmill. The exercises are the same. You're just at different levels. For now, anyway.

Here's the barebones breakdown of these three phases, which I designed along with one of the leading personal trainers in the country—Joseph Dowdell, a certified strength and conditioning specialist through the National Strength and Conditioning Association, and the owner of Peak Performance gym in New York City. Joe has worked out everyone from top pro athletes to actresses and runway models.

- Phase I: **PRIMING THE PUMP!** This prepares you for the rigors of my training style.
- Phase II: **FUELING THE FIRE!** The emphasis here becomes burning fat and building muscle with which to sculpt.
- Phase III: **MAXING IT OUT!** Lean out to showcase and sculpt your new-found muscle, while making further improvements in strength and power.

This six- or 12-week scheme, depending on your fitness level, allows you to build by starting off with simple lifts and body-weight moves in Phase I; moving on to more demanding moves in Phase II; and then adding some instability elements while shortening rest periods in Phase III, at which point you're training more or less like I do. Over the course of these six weeks, I'll gradually build up your strength and conditioning while introducing you to different "qualities" of training, especially power and explosiveness. Those qualities aren't just for guys, either. You need them if you want to smash a tennis ball or spike a volleyball, ladies. And I'll do it in a way that's safe, effective, and most of all, fun.

All of your fitness your goals are going to be satisfied without you even telling me what they are, because we're going to hit every single area of your body to the max. No stone will be left unturned. If you want to have a great butt, you're going to have a great butt at the end of this program, even though you didn't tell me you wanted a great butt. Ditto for firm arms, a tight stomach, and every other showcase body part. About the only thing I can't guarantee is a set of dimples like mine!

That's because these aren't your run-of-the-mill, garden-variety, blah-blah-blah workouts. Not even. Cookie cutters belong in the kitchen, not in the gym. Normally, you don't see many people doing bench jumps. You don't seem them doing a set of bench presses followed by medicine ball tosses. Or triple sets that include weight moves and jumping jacks. Or basketball, volleyball, or dance workouts in between their gym workouts. Uniqueness and variability are two of your watchwords over the next six or 12 weeks. That's why experienced gym goers and newbies alike will grow muscle and melt fat using this program.

Not all of you are starting off in the kind of shape displayed on the cover of this book, and that doesn't matter a lick. Like I said, over *20 years* I've worked really hard to bring my body to this level of development and conditioning. But use that image as motivation. That's why it's there. In fact, if you're a beginner, you have an even bigger window of opportunity through which to make rapid gains than other people do. Consider: At this point, you're nowhere close to your potential. If you've been training for a while, and you're already at 90 percent of your potential, it's a lot harder to reach 95 percent than it is for someone at 50 percent to reach 75 percent. The increases in your progress are so much smaller and slower if you're already in the 90s. You're already so close to the top of your mountain. If you're just starting out, I envy what lies ahead you for. Be excited about that prospect, not intimidated by it.

Everything in this book is modular, turnkey, and fun—especially the sports sessions, which you won't find anywhere else. The workouts can be followed to the letter yet adapted to your individual needs and goals. As we proceed, I'll also explain how these phases can be expanded as needed over the next 6 or 12 weeks. Maybe your primary objective isn't leaning out, but gaining muscle. In that case, I'll explain how to shift the emphasis from cuts to a fuller muscle tone. The reverse holds true as well: If you're already as muscular as you want to be, but you want sculpt what you possess, and become leaner along the way, I'll demonstrate how to do that as well. Throughout, I'll also show you how to use the gym workouts to improve your sports performance, and vice versa.

Along the way, every workout in this book is designed to promote balanced development, because symmetry looks good and prevent injuries for men and women alike. I'll be the first to admit that at certain times in the past, I've been as guilty as the next person of focusing on chest and arms—beach muscles, they call 'em—to the detriment of the rest of my body. (For you women, maybe it's spending half your training session working the butt blaster. Same basic idea, right?) Indeed, I'm blessed with good DNA for developing strong arms and a big chest. My dad worked a sledgehammer for the city for decades, and his grip clamps down like a vice. When I was a kid, I would shake his hand, and suddenly *squeeze* it as hard as I could. He couldn't feel a thing. To this day, my dad could still squash my hand if he wanted to (not that he ever would, of course!). Not surprisingly, when I train arms and chest today, they sprout like weeds shooting up through those sidewalks my dad pounds into submission using his jackhammer.

I can thank my father for that, but I now realize that being a fit and athletic person means training your entire body, not just the parts that you feel like training. If possible, I like hitting everything, everywhere in a single workout. Not ignoring legs, for example. I like feeling every muscle in my body nice and tight. One-stop shopping for an amazing body.

Everyone who follows this program will achieve a dramatically improved fitness level. Your overall conditioning will be much higher. You'll be able to do *work* for longer periods of time because your endurance will have improved. You'll also notice a marked change in body composition: more lean mass, better muscle tone, less body fat. Combine those three elements, and you won't just be stopping traffic, ladies—you'll be sending it into reverse as guys crane their neck to check you out. What's more, expect improvements, perhaps dramatic ones, in your maximum strength and power. I'm talking 25 to 30 percent over six weeks for some of you.

Reflecting that, the basic framework is lifting weights and cardio three days a week. On two or three other days in a given week, you'll be performing sports-based activities that tie in smartly with those gym workouts. Above all, I like mixing it up when I bust a workout. I do a lot of different things, and I'll try pretty much everything once. I'm a big fan of surprising my body every day with something a little bit different. It does for my body what hosting does for my brain. When you never know what's coming your way, you have to stay on your toes.

That also explains the rationale behind the 10-minute workouts scattered throughout the book. These are

HEY, MARIO!

What should I be drinking while I'm following your workout program?

Except for milk, drink beverages that add little or nothing to your daily calorie count. Water is the obvious option, but zero-calorie coffee and its fat-burning caffeine works, too, as long as you don't exceed three cups per day. Teas (hot or cold, black or green) are another great option that enhances fat burning without adding calories. I'm less bullish on diet sodas and other diet drinks, but they're okay.

separate from the main workouts, and they reflect as simple truth: Days will come when you don't have even 45 minutes to work out. When that happens, these mini-workouts can serve as super-fast but super-effective substitutes. They're what I use a lot when I'm traveling, or on a set that happens to have a workout trailer or some weights and maybe a treadmill scattered around.

Underlying the main program, though, are weight workouts in the gym (a.k.a., resistance training) and cardiovascular exercise (a.k.a., cardio). We're building a structure—your body, in this case—and those two elements form the foundation. You can't shape up, and you certainly can't finish this program, if you don't train both your skeletal muscles and the most important muscle of all: your ticker. Even if you've jogged but never lifted a dumbbell in your whole life, I need you to weight train along with working the cardio machines. Weights rule! It's not a macho thing; it's what exercise scientists know works the best for growing muscle and burning fat.

If you don't believe me, read the latest research from a group of University of Connecticut researchers. They took a group of overweight subjects, pegged their diet to 1,500 calories a day, and then divided them among three groups. Those who did cardio and weights shed considerably more fat than both a cardio-only group and those who didn't lift a finger. That's even truer with my program, because my weight workouts are really like cardio workouts.

Other workout books take one of two approaches to weight training: *old-school* training vs. *functional* training. I'll explain both approaches in a moment, but perhaps the one and only thing shared by both camps is an intense aversion to the other camp's approach. I disagree; I believe both approaches possess merits and drawbacks. The unique thing about my approach to weight training is that I combine elements of each camp. Call it the best of both worlds.

As the name implies, old-school training hearkens back decades, to the very beginnings of bodybuilding, a sport in which male and female athletes alike are judged based on their muscle, symmetry and conditioning. The idea here is that the human body comprises a vary array of muscles, all of which must be developed in harmony to create a balanced, aesthetically pleasing body.

This is how one of my heroes, Arnold, trained. (No last name needed, right?) While this bodybuilding-style approach takes advantage of squats, bench presses, and other exercises that recruit a whole host of muscles in order to move a weight, other exercises from the old school zero in on individual, smaller muscles, even the teeniest, tiniest ones. A seated calf raise is designed to work only calves. A barbell curl is designed to work only biceps. A cable pushdown is meant to train only triceps. In fact, the people who do these exercises will tell you that the more you isolate these smaller muscles, the better you're doing. According to them, if you're trying to work your triceps, you *don't* want your chest or shoulders pitching in to help. Because they're bigger and stronger, these muscles have a tendency to take over. If you took this approach to the absolute limit of human muscular development by aspiring to become Mr. or Ms. Olympia, bodybuilding judges would slash your score because your physique lacked symmetry, defined according to archetypes that Greek sculptors chiseled from marble.

Let's call the old-school trainers and athletes the *isolationists*.

The functional-training crowd dismisses the isolationists as dinosaurs out of touch with the latest advances of modern training science. They would like nothing more than to take many of those old-school exercises and toss them out once and for all. They argue that this isn't the way you use your body in the real world, so you shouldn't train it like that in the gym, either. The functional crowd sees no need to target specific muscles. For them, everything boils down to taking those actions that your body does repeatedly as part of everyday life—stepping, pushing, pulling, squatting, and rotating—and replicating them in the gym, only with resistance or some other challenge applied.

As a result, functional trainers employ barbells and dumbbells, but only for certain exercises. Most of them have never met a workout machine they liked. (As one trainer once told me, Smith machines are useful for one thing only: hanging laundry out to dry.) What they *really* like are pushups, chinups, and other exercises that use the body as a weight. If they do use an apparatus, it's likely to be rope for climbing up or jumping over, Russian kettle bells for hoisting around, or medicine balls for throwing against a wall or to a partner. Put these trainers in a junkyard or a cluttered attic, and they'd have no trouble coming up with a challenging workout.

Let's call the modern-school trainers and athletes the *integrationists*.

While some aspects of old-school training should be cast aside, and others need updating, I *love* training old school, the way Arnold did. I believe devoutly that it still provides benefits that the integrationists can't match with their newfangled ways. I don't think my body could look the way I want it to look, the way it does look, without heaping helpings of some of these traditional bodybuilding moves. What's more, I think the functional crowd goes overboard in its preoccupation with stability and balance. Stabilization work is important, without question; yet in placing *so* much emphasis there, they really compromise muscle and strength development. The clients of these trainers never make too many actual gains in strength because all they're doing is stability, stability, stability. Unfortunately, the central nervous system fatigues before the body really has the chance to move enough weight to activate most of a muscle's fibers. It's not the most advantageous way to improve muscle tone, strength, and power.

Having said that, I like the way the isolationists mix and free-weight and machine moves. Free weights force you to recruit more helper muscles for balance and control. Free weights also allow your body to call the shots and stay in charge of the exercise. In contrast, one limitation with certain machines is that the path simply is what it is. For instance, on a machine version of the bench press, the machine will perform the move exactly the same way whether I'm pushing the weight, you're pushing the weight, or a guy who stands six-foot-eight is pushing the weight. Yet if we did a bench press with free weights, your body would send them in one pathway, and mine would send it in another. Now we're both moving the way our bodies were designed to, rather than being locked into a groove.

I love dumbbells, and you'll be picking them up frequently as you work your way through my program. What's great about them is that they require even

9 REASONS TO KEEP A TRAINING JOURNAL

1) Instead of thinking, *What should I do at the gym today?* you can review your recent workouts. Hone in on what you hope to accomplish this particular session.

2) You'll remain aware of the importance of every single workout. Each one is a brick in the building that you're constructing.

3) When you write down an upcoming workout, that visualization process can get you pumped to the right level of intensity and focus.

4) As you check off items from your list during the workout, you'll gain a head of steam by systematically knocking off smaller tasks en route to a killer workout.

5) Research shows that writing down a task increases the likelihood of completing it from 20 percent to more than 90 percent! I put everything in my little PDA, so I have little reminders, but a notebook and pen work just as well.

6) Especially for someone who has worked out for a long time, boredom can become public enemy number one. Staring at your goals—or your stagnation—in black and white forces you to keep challenging yourself.

7) As you write and read, you'll pay attention not only to how you look, but also to how you feel. That'll give you even more motivation to stick with the program.

8) Only by keeping a journal will you begin to see patterns and repetitions emerging. Maybe your Monday workouts, which always happen late at night, are improving, but your Friday workouts are stuck in neutral. Perhaps you should hold off on those sessions until later.

9) A periodic shot of confidence. Viewed daily or weekly, improvements can be almost imperceptible. Looking back over months, you'll be surprised—maybe even amazed—at just how much progress you've made.

more helper muscles than barbells. I also think that over time they produce slightly fuller and more complete development than barbells, especially around your all-important joints. You can't necessarily train as heavy with dumbbells as you can with barbells, but for women, especially, I don't believe that super-heavy weights are more beneficial than moderate weights. The important thing is to concentrate on controlling the movement. Leave the gorilla stuff for offensive lineman and moving-and-storage guys.

Also, the pathway of movement is even more natural, and the range of motion greater, with dumbbells than it is with barbells. At the top of either a bench press or a military press, for example, you can bring your arms toward each other, something you can't do with a barbell. Suddenly, you're telling the weights where to go, controlling the actions of each wrist, coordinating how and when to squeeze each chest muscle—all the while making sure to move the weights up and down at the same speed. You basically develop your own style of training with dumbbells. Another advantage: It makes it easier to do the workouts at home if you're so inclined. (By the way, if you find that you have a strong preference for either dumbbells or barbells, trust your instincts. Where you see, say, a "dumbbell squat" listed in the workout program, feel free to perform a barbell squat instead. I won't hold it against you.)

But the attitude that free weights are for serious training, while machines are for sissies, doesn't hold any water with me. Stimulating a muscle means performing the right move with correct form, whether it's with dumbbells, a barbell, machines, cables, or a can of tomato soup, for that matter. There are exceptions, like the aforementioned bench press, but used correctly, some machines do work just as well as free weights. In certain cases, they actually represent the preferred option. If the resistance is sufficient to stimulate growth, and you're taking the load through a full range of motion, it doesn't much matter if you're pushing a free-floating hunk of iron or the mechanical arms of a machine. It's all good.

Just ask my trainer, Jimmy Peña. "Especially nowadays, with so many companies making so many sophisticated machines, there's no reason not to use

HEY, MARIO!
What's the simplest way to curb my appetite?

Chew sugarless gum. British researchers did an experiment in which some subjects chomped on sugarless gum for 15 minutes per hour, and some didn't. The gum smackers consumed 36 fewer calories, on average, when working their way through a snack table three hours later. Chew gum at the stove, too. You'll be less likely to taste-test along the way.

every tool at your disposal," says Jimmy. "Resistance is resistance, and when it comes to building muscle, it's all good." He knows of what he speaks: Jimmy was formerly strength and conditioning coordinator at the Baylor-Tom Landry Sports Science and Research Center in Dallas; then became the fitness director at The Ritz-Carlton hotel in Half Moon Bay, California; now serves as fitness director of *Muscle & Fitness* magazine; and has been certified by the National Strength and Conditioning Association as a strength and conditioning specialist, the gold standard in the field.

Machines are great for isolating your target muscles. If you've suffered an injury to, say, your lower back or knees, certain machines can actually be safer than their free-weight counterparts. A lot of the new machines they're coming up with these days really work wonders. Even a lot of the basic moves such as barbell rows and deadlifts now have effective machine counterparts. It's also easier for a spotter to help you with assisted reps on a machine version of, say, a heaving rowing movement for back, as opposed to the free-weight version.

The bottom line: Mix it up! Depending on what gym I'm training at, I like to use a variety of exercises. Within the same workout, I combine dumbbells, barbells, machines, and cable moves, and that's just for starters. If I'm training chest, I might bounce back and forth between the cable stacks, for crossovers; the pec deck, for machine flyes; and dumbbells, for flyes. It all depends on how I'm feeling that day.

So while I disagree with certain aspects of functional training and believe its advocates dismiss bodybuilding-style training too quickly and casually, the integrationists do champion some training strategies that I like a lot. For example, functional training prepares you well for hitting the court, ring, or playing field. Whether you box, play flag football, run pickup hoops, or dance the samba in front of 20 million television viewers, your body has to recruit muscles in new and unpredictable ways. I hit the gym regularly and box competitively, but when I appeared on *Dancing with the Stars*, I would wake up feeling sore in so many weird places. Take my lower back: I was really surprised at how much that hurt. It was killing me! After a day of rehearsals, I felt like I had been digging a ditch on a chain gang all day.

So the functional training, courtesy of the integrationists, is here so you can play and compete like me. The old school, bodybuilding-style training, courtesy of the isolationists, is here so you can look like me.

Along with hitting the weights, you'll be doing some serious cardiovascular exercise over the next 6 or 12 weeks. Forewarned is forearmed, however: You may find it completely different from your current cardio regimen, and perhaps even different from any cardio you've done before. Staying with the theme that change keeps your body guessing and adapting, I ask you to switch between different cardio machines as the program unfolds. Each machine forces you to use different muscle groups in new ways.

More important, instead of running or biking in the gym or outside at the same steady pace for a certain length of time, you're going to be training interval-style. You'll love it, trust me. Interval training is very much like my resistance-training workouts, or my boxing training, for that matter: quick, super-intense bursts of activity, then downshifting for a brief period, then another burst, and so on—boom, boom, boom! Intervals are just what the doctor ordered if your endurance training makes you feel like a robot these days. Do 15 minutes of those, and you'll leave the gym smoked, with a better workout under your belt than the guy over in the corner who's been jogging at the same place for an hour while reading *The Wall Street Journal*.

Unfortunately, cardiovascular exercise has become the most boring part of training for many people. That's a shame, because it actually offers the greatest potential for improvisation and fun. Whereas intervals in a boxing match or basketball game are unpredictable, interval cardio works best when planned down to the second. The hard part, the time when you're working really hard, is called the *work* portion. The easier part, the time when you downshift, or perhaps stop working altogether, is called the *rest* portion (although the rest is usually better thought of as *active rest*—like walking instead of sprinting on a treadmill). Over time, various aspects of an interval program can be altered: the ratio between *rest* and *work*; the intensity level of the *work* portion; or the duration of the entire session.

Interval training exercises your heart, as do other forms of cardio, but its biggest advantage over steady-state exercise concerns the almost supernatural way in which it melts away lard. Intervals create something called "metabolic disturbance," a term relayed to me by Joseph Dowdell. That sounds alarming, but it's actually a good thing. In a recent Australian study, people who cranked out 20 minutes of high-intensity interval training three days a week said bye-bye to 10 percent of their body fat. Those who slogged through 40 minutes of steady cardio? They still had the same love handles and saddlebags to show for their antiquated approach to cardio.

The advantages aren't limited to fat burning, however. Intervals also . . .

● Improve cardiovascular fitness dramatically. One result: When you're training or playing a sport, your endurance will be better.
● Raise levels of the HDL cholesterol—the kind the keeps your arteries from becoming clogged.

- Decrease the number of times the heart beats per minute, which contributes to long-term heart health.
- Save time. I don't know about you, but I'm busy, and 10 to 15 minutes beats the heck out of 60 minutes every time. Intervals can be exhausting, but they're quick. That allows you to integrate cardio with weights in ways that would be nearly impossible with more conventional endurance training. Try spending an hour on the treadmill and then lifting afterward. Good luck with that. Forget for a moment about the physical fatigue. Your brain would be too zonked for you to go hit the weights.

One way to measure cardiovascular fitness is through a measurement called VO_2 max. I'm not an exercise scientist, so I'll let Abbie I. Smith, a master's candidate in exercise physiology at the University of Oklahoma, who I interviewed for this book, explain: "VO_2 max measures the maximum amount of oxygen you can consume. When you're huffing and puffing on the treadmill, you're sucking in oxygen and expelling carbon dioxide. With someone who's out of shape, the maximum amount of oxygen they can consume is going to occur very early. Intervals are great at increasing that threshold."

Another nice thing about intervals is that they're very sports specific. The work-to-rest ratios will vary from sport to sport, and from play to play within each sport, but it's the same basic principle: none of us moves at the same pace all the time. That's why endurance athletes who grind out miles after mile on the road or on a treadmill will start sucking wind as soon as they join a pick-up basketball game.

Because interval training is so efficient, I can combine it with my weight session, which is how I like to train. To me, weights and cardio complement each other. Some people think either/or; I think both. Science has my back on this one, too. For example, wind sprint workouts—which are essentially intervals taken outdoors—work your lungs but also strengthen your lower body strength, according to a group of Croatian researchers. In one recent study, those who replaced their weekly weight workouts with three high-intensity cardio sessions increased their leg strength by 10 percent, an impressive accomplishment given that the time span was only 10 weeks.

As if that isn't enough, in each phase, I add in two of my favorite sports activities to augment the gym training, and explain how specific things I do in the gym help those activities, and vice versa. In my world, in-the-gym training and on-the-field athletics constitute one giant, synergistic feedback loop. Researchers have found that people tend to participate in sports because they're fun; *that* fact, in and of itself, motivates them keep playing whatever their particular game or sport. On the other hand, researchers find that to stick it out in the gym over time, most people need external motivation: the promise of a better body, improved health—something that lies outside of their current experience. In other words, if you play baseball, and all you derive from it is the enjoyment of playing the game—you don't look any different for having done so—you probably would do it anyway. However, if you worked out in the gym, and it didn't make you look any different, you probably would drop it soon enough. That motivational difference is huge, and it explains this book's unique merger of gym workouts and sports training.

In fact, researchers at the University of Michigan found that women are *way* better about exercising when their motivation is simply enjoyment, as opposed to turning their body into that of a chiseled, sculpted goddess. I would be shocked if the same division didn't apply to men. That makes it a little harder to stick with a workout program consisting only of weights and cardiovascular exercise. So by adding these sports activities to the regimen, I'm helping you build more muscle, burn more body fat, and stick with the program for the long haul.

Finally, this workout book contains extensive guidance on nutritional support, including 21 daily plans—7 days' worth for each phase! This is like a pyramid, with training one side, the mental aspect on another, and nutrition on another. If only one side is weak, the structure won't maintain its integrity. It's no good to hit the gym for these amazing workouts if you're not going to give your body the nutritional support it needs to recover, repair, and rebuild.

Phase 1 Weeks 1 and 2

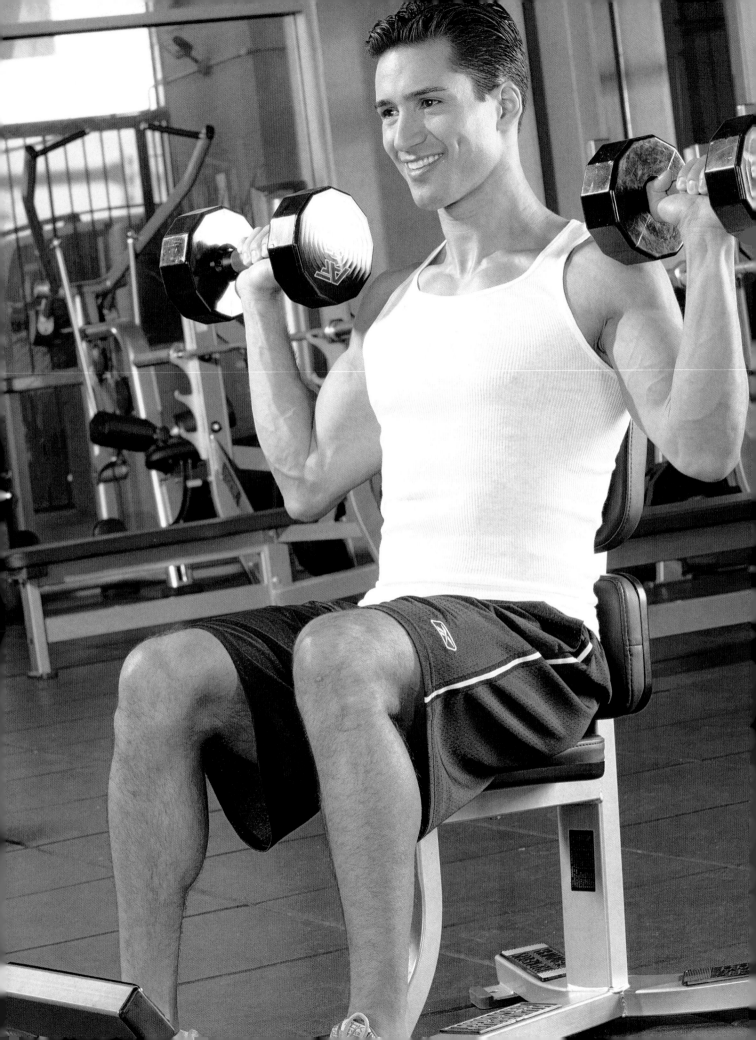

2 Priming the Pump!

Are you ready? Let's bust a workout.

For you to train exactly like I do now would feel like taking a swan dive into ice water. You would experience a shock to your system, and you probably wouldn't want to experience that feeling again. To avoid that shock, I've designed these first two weeks of the program to ease you into training. If you already have some training experience in the gym, I want you to perform these workouts for two weeks. If you're a complete newbie, stay in this phase for four weeks. You need to spend a little more time preparing your body for the increased demands in intensity that will follow.

If you're chomping at the bit from having to spend twice as long in this phase as someone else, take heart: You'll be making increasing progress the entire time you're in it. Those of you whose training experience places you above that level can move out more quickly because you're going to need more and different stimuli. The real benefits of weight training accrue gradually over time; nothing, except maybe injuries, happens overnight, regardless of how impatient you are.

The backbone of this book is the workout charts. As you encounter them, you'll come across terminology that is essential to unlocking a better body. Let's review them before we pick up that first weight. Consider this your first warm up.

Exercise Selection: You'll be doing two exercises together in this phase, with the pairings going from upper to lower body according to a technique called *supersetting* (more on that in a minute). The exercises have been carefully selected to maximize your initial results. Exercises such as the dumbbell split squat and pushup—the first pairing—are called multi-joint, or compound, exercises. As the name suggests, executing them requires more than one set of joints working together. For example, on the split squat, your hips, knees, and ankles are all involved. On the pushup, your shoulders, elbows, and wrists all need to get into the action.

These "big" moves hit major muscles (legs and chest, respectively), but when done correctly, they work nearly the entire body, not only building muscle but also burning fat. I can't overemphasize the importance of these exercises. Canadian researchers found that performing poorly in a pushup test makes someone 78 percent more likely to gain 20 pounds of flab over the next two decades. That's because training big muscles really stokes the fat-burning fires.

Sets and Supersets: One of the best ways to make your workouts more efficient is with a technique called supersetting, which is used extensively in this book. It involves doing one exercise immediately after the next without resting in between moves, other than the time it takes to move from one apparatus to another. After completing one such superset, you rest briefly and then—*boom*—repeat.

Ideally, the two body parts being paired in a superset should perform opposing functions. Supersets can also be done on the same body part, called compound sets. Biceps and triceps, quads and hamstrings, chest and back—they're all classic superset pairings. For example, your chest helps push things away from your torso; your back, particularly your lats, helps to pull things toward you. Even though your entire body is taxed any time you do an intense set, the opposing muscle group can relax somewhat as you train its counterpart. At the most fundamental level, supersetting any two body parts means

HEY, MARIO!
What's the best time of day for me to hit the gym?
Whenever you'll actually show up. Sure, there are niggling differences between day and night. A study in the *Journal of Athletic Training* found that a person's balance peaks at 10 a.m.—which might help with my trickier exercises—and then drops off. But blood flow peaks in the afternoon, which is a workout plus, and another study found that swimmers peaked 11:00 p.m. Don't worry about when you go. **Just go.**

taking the normal rest periods for each and folding them into the working sets of the opposing muscle group. Supersetting is one of the secrets to juggling a vigorous workout regimen with a demanding schedule like mine. A workout that might otherwise take 60 minutes suddenly takes 30, with no loss of effectiveness.

Repetition: A *repetition*, or rep, means taking an exercise from start to finish. Take a dumbbell, raise it up to your shoulder, and then lower it back to where it started, and you've just completed one rep of a dumbbell curl. The *positive* (concentric) half of a rep is where you're fighting against gravity. Here, that would be the raising of the dumbbell up toward your shoulder. The *negative* (eccentric) portion involves lowering the weight. The only battle here is with gravity—making sure the weight doesn't just free-fall. You need to control it in both directions to prevent injury and gain the full effectiveness of the move.

Often, you'll see the reps given as a range, not as a single number. Pullups, for example, are listed in Phase I at 12 to 15 reps. So it's okay to do 12, 13, 14, or 15 reps—but not 11 or 16. This range determines the weight you pick up off the rack at the gym, or the place you stick the pin in the cable stack. The load should be light enough for you to reach the low end of the rep range, yet heavy enough that you can't exceed the upper limit. Once you can exceed this

6 REASONS YOU NEED 8 HOURS OF SLEEP

1) Tossing and turning can make you fat. Researchers at the University of Chicago found that lack of sleep revs up our hunger hormones. Canadian sleep researchers found that sleeping five to six hours a night makes you 69 percent more likely to gain excess poundage than those who slumber for the full eight.

2) If you don't snooze, and then booze, you lose. Impaired sleep heightens the effect of alcohol on your body, making you much more likely to have an accident.

3) Diabetes loves insomnia almost as much as sugar. Less sleep reduces your body's ability to metabolize glucose.

4) Sleeplessness takes a toll on your ticker. Researchers at the University of California at San Diego found that even healthy men who wake up in the middle of the night are more likely to suffer a heart attack.

5) Pillow talk is great; mumbling in your sleep isn't. If you talk in your sleep more than three or four times a week, see a sleep specialist, stat.

6) Lack of sleep depresses your immune system. As a result, you'll be more prone to colds, upper-respiratory-tract infections, and other illnesses that'll keep you out of the gym.

limit, switch to a slightly heavier weight. (Five pounds is a good increment to advance for most people.) In order to make a muscle bigger, it needs to overcome a certain amount of resistance. As the weights become heavier, your muscles become stronger and larger to compensate. I've certainly gotten a lot stronger over the years—as you become older, you develop that "man" strength that young guys don't have. Just to cite one example, the most I could bench then was 225, but now I can do 305. And my body reflects that improvement in strength.

Form: The key to getting the most from this workout is performing each of the exercises with better form than you've ever used before—even though supersetting makes cheating all the more tempting! If following these exercise descriptions to the letter requires you to use less weight than you did previously, don't be discouraged by that adjustment. You're on the right track. You're probably getting more out of those exercises than you ever have before.

Strict form means maintaining a sound body position that keeps the majority of the emphasis on the working muscles and decreases the chances of an injury. The workout photos were shot with precise detail so that you'll know exactly what constitutes a "sound position" for every exercise I ask you to perform. One of my favorite tricks for keeping my form nice and tight is thinking in terms of working muscles, rather than in terms of lifting weights. During any set—regardless of what exercise it is—try to really *feel* the muscles working. If you don't feel them, something's wrong.

Don't assume you're using proper technique just because you haven't suffered an injury yet. I've heard people say, "Dude, I reached down to lift a box in my garage, and suddenly my back gave out. I haven't been able to roll over in bed for three days." News flash: Your lower back didn't just lock up suddenly without warning. More likely, incorrect lifting form over the years has inflicted major damage. Lifting that box was the straw that broke the camel's back—no pun intended.

How does a person reach that point? At gyms around the country, you'll find wannabes arching their backs and using momentum to swing weights up and past the trickiest moments in the lift, called *sticking points.* They clearly don't know what they're doing, and they just make up stuff! I'm not one to interfere with them—unless they ask, of course—but it makes me cringe every time I witness it. You never want to see someone hurt himself.

"Cheating," as this practice is otherwise known, allows a muscle to handle more than it could if you were using strict technique. Seeing people toss around big hunks of iron, you might be tempted to think, *Hey, if a little body English has made them big and muscular, maybe it'll work for me.* Don't do it. When you can no longer complete a rep using strict form, set the weights down. The set is now O-V-E-R. Period. It's a wrap. Wait till you can properly lift another set.

Cardio: At the end of each weight session during this phase, you'll go straight to interval-style cardiovascular training. Why after instead of before? Research has shown that resistance training and all of its benefits are compromised if preceded by cardio. The only time I would recommend doing cardio first is if that's the only time you *can* do it.

Warming Up: Practically from the first time we lift a pacifier, we're told to stretch thoroughly right before working out. But as you read this book, you're going to learn that a lot of things you've doing in the gym your entire life have been wrong—dead wrong. And this is one of them. You do want to warm up first by elevating your body temperature with five minutes or so on a treadmill or stationary bike. But the best time to stretch is *after* your weight workout ends, when your muscle tissue is warm and elastic.

What's the point in trying to stretch cold muscle tissue that's brittle and prone to pulls and tears? What's more, stretching directly before a workout actually *decreases* the amount of force those muscles can generate, by about 15 percent, according to researchers from the United Kingdom. If you must stretch before training, do it 15 to 30 minutes before the workout, not immediately beforehand.

Abs: Finally, before I usher you into the gym, let me say a few words about abs. Heck, the A word is probably what some of you were after when you bought this book in the first place. Surprise, surprise—you perform only one dedicated abs move during Phase I. Yes, I train my abs. I train them intensely. Note that I said *intensely*—not endlessly, nor even for a particularly long time, at least by some people's standards. It doesn't take long to train abs,

HEY, MARIO!

What should I do after an exhausting set of intervals—keep walking, rather than bending over with my hands on my knees?

Neither! If you're spent, lie down for 5 or even 10 minutes, despite what every sports coach has been drumming into your head since Little League. A recent study in the *Journal of Applied Physiology* found that cyclists who flopped on their backs produced twice as much sweat and slowed their heart rate faster than those who sat upright. Instead of pooling in the muscles you just worked, blood flows more easily back to the heart.

partly because the muscles of your core fire first in every exercise. All the force that you exert originates in your torso; only then is it transferred through your arms and legs. I also train my lower back as much as my abs, which balances out and injury-proofs my midsection. Once you hurt your back, it will always be vulnerable.

Guys want to make their abs pop, and girls want a flat tummy. Guess what? The same training strategies and diet tips produce both results. (Hormonal differences account for differences in how much the abdominal muscles protrude.) Remember that it's not how many crunches you do, it's the amount of body fat between the skin and the muscle. People who are overweight have abs. Skinny people have abs. Everyone in between has abs of some sort. Abdominal definition is simply a reflection of how well-developed the ab muscles are, and whether you can see them.

The core work you perform in Workouts A and B during Phase I will help when you reach the running part of Workout D. Strengthening the core muscles heightens the connection between the upper and lower body so that when you run, the knee lift and arm swing are synchronized. That gives you explosive power. Next thing you know, you'll be sprinting like Jose Reyes taking off for second base.

Finally, as you prepare to start changing your body and changing your life, keep in mind that fat-loss programs like this aren't all-or-nothing propositions. Even if you don't stick with the program 100 percent of the time, you're still going to achieve positive results by completing part of it. You will be headed in the right direction. *How quickly* you arrive there is less important than the fact that you *will* arrive there eventually.

PHASE I PRIMARY GOALS:

- Muscular endurance
- Core strength endurance
- Improved flexibility

Phase I

Beginner							
	Monday	Tuesday	Wednesday	Thursday	Friday	Saturday	Sunday
WEEK 1:	Workout A	Rest	Workout B	Rest	Workout A	Workout C	Rest
WEEK 2:	Workout B	Rest	Workout A	Rest	Workout B	Workout D	Rest
WEEK 3:	Workout A	Rest	Workout B	Rest	Workout A	Workout C	Rest
WEEK 4:	Workout B	Rest	Workout A	Rest	Workout B	Workout D	Rest
Intermediate and Advanced							
	Monday	Tuesday	Wednesday	Thursday	Friday	Saturday	Sunday
WEEK 1:	Workout A	Rest	Workout B	Workout C	Workout A	Workout D	Rest
WEEK 2:	Workout B	Rest	Workout A	Workout C	Workout B	Workout D	Rest

While fitness programs offer amazing benefits, they do place stress on the human body. Please see your doctor before beginning this program if you have doubts about your ability to handle these workouts—especially if you have any history of heart disease or other cardiovascular problems. Also, before practicing the exercises in this book, be sure that your equipment is well-maintained, and do not take risks beyond your level of experience. Better safe than sorry!

Phase I:
Workout A

Sequence	Week	Exercise	Sets[1]	Reps[2]	Rest[3]
A1	1	Dumbbell Split Squat	3	10–12/side	↓
	2	Dumbbell Split Squat	3	10–12/side	↓
	3	Dumbbell Split Squat	3	10–12/side	↓
	4	Dumbbell Split Squat	3	10–12/side	↓
A2	1	Pushup	3	↑20	60
	2	Pushup	3	↑20	60
	3	Pushup	3	↑20	60
	4	Pushup	3	↑20	60
B1	1	Hip Bridge	3	10–12	↓
	2	Hip Bridge	3	10–12	↓
	3	Hip Bridge	3	10–12	↓
	4	Hip Bridge	3	10–12	↓
B2	1	Pullup (Assisted) or Pulldown	3	12–15	60
	2	Pullup (Assisted) or Pulldown	3	12–15	60
	3	Pullup (Assisted) or Pulldown	3	12–15	60
	4	Pullup (Assisted) or Pulldown	3	12–15	60
C1	1	Speed Skating Drill	3	12–15/side	↓
	2	Speed Skating Drill	3	12–15/side	↓
	3	Speed Skating Drill	3	12–15/side	↓
	4	Speed Skating Drill	3	12–15/side	↓
C2	1	Seated Dumbbell Curl/Shoulder Press	3	12–15	60
	2	Seated Dumbbell Curl/Shoulder Press	3	12–15	60
	3	Seated Dumbbell Curl/Shoulder Press	3	12–15	60
	4	Seated Dumbbell Curl/Shoulder Press	3	12–15	60
D1	1	Reverse Crunch	3	10–12	60
	2	Reverse Crunch	3	10–12	60
	3	Reverse Crunch	3	10–12	60
	4	Reverse Crunch	3	10–12	60
E1		Perform lateral hop intervals. Do 6–8 reps of 20–30 seconds of hops, followed by 60–90 seconds of easy jogging in place.			

[1] Do modified supersets with each pair of exercises listed with the same number (for example, A1 and A2); that is, do the prescribed number of sets for each of the two exercises in alternating fashion before moving on to the next pairing. (For example, if the program calls for three sets, do one set of split squats followed by one set of push-ups, and then repeat twice). Rest in between each set as indicated.

[2] The last rep you can finish with complete control and perfect form should fall within this range, so select your weight accordingly. Once you have completed all your repetitions with your current weight for two consecutive workouts, increase your poundage slightly. Five pounds for each new step is a good rule of thumb.

[3] Between supersets, measured in seconds.

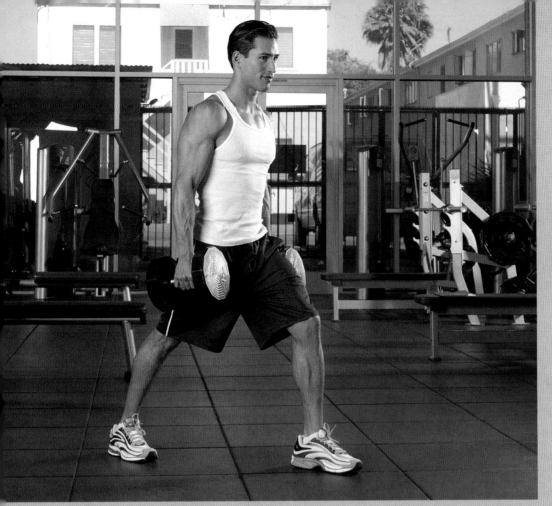

DUMBBELL SPLIT SQUAT

Great for:
football,
tae kwon do

Get ready!

Hold dumbbells at arm's length, palms facing each other. Place your feet in a "scissors" configuration: one in front of the other, both flat on the floor.

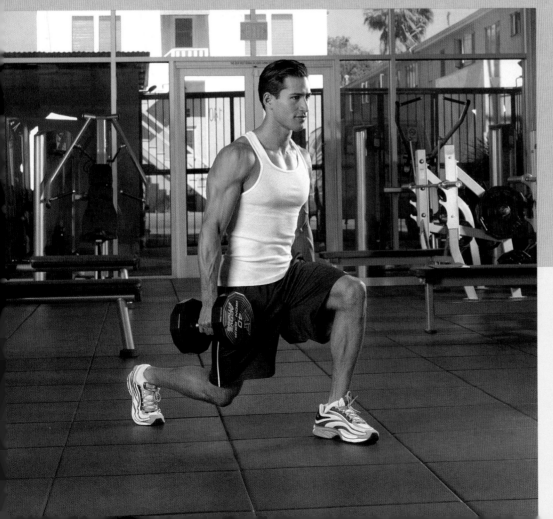

Go!

Keeping your torso erect, bend both knees to descend. Near the bottom, your rear knee should almost touch the floor. Immediately push yourself back up to the starting position. Do the same number of reps with each leg.

Watch out for:

Your knee joint shaking side to side as you move up and down. If this happens you probably need to trade those dumbbells for a lighter pair.

23

PUSHUP

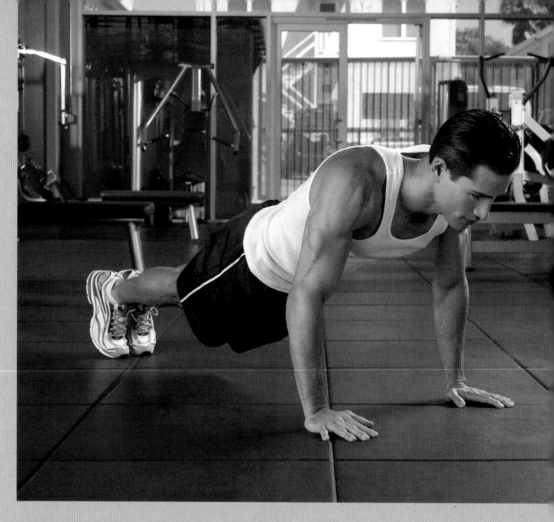

Get ready!

Assume the standard pushup position: (A) hands on the floor in line with your shoulders, but spaced slightly wider than shoulder-width apart; and (B) legs straightened behind you. Your body should resemble a plank from head to heels.

Go!

Bend your elbows to lower your torso until your chest nearly touches the floor. Push yourself back up to the starting position.

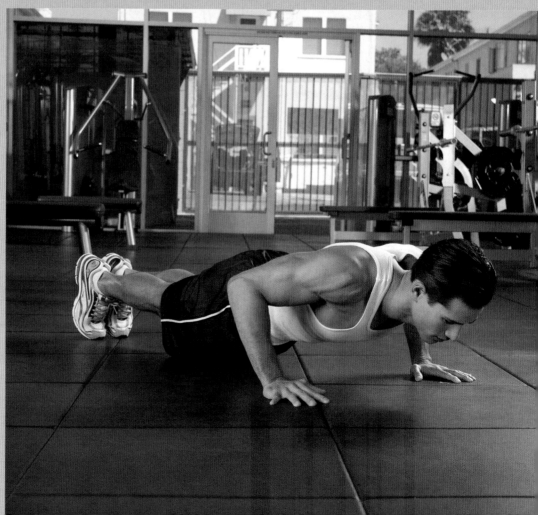

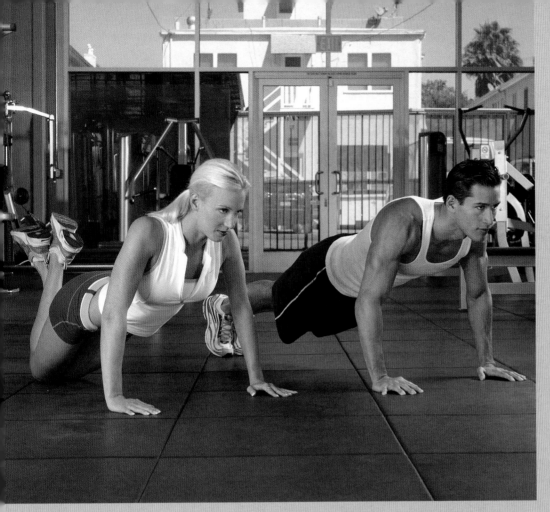

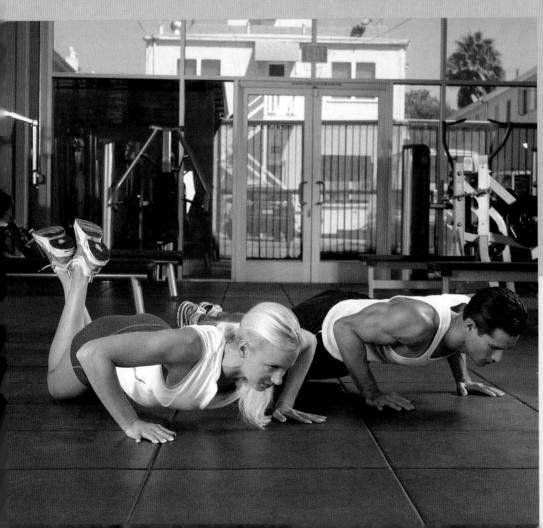

Tweak:

If you can't do enough regular pushups, rest your knees on the floor. The move should now be easier, allowing you to complete the desired number of reps.

HIP BRIDGE

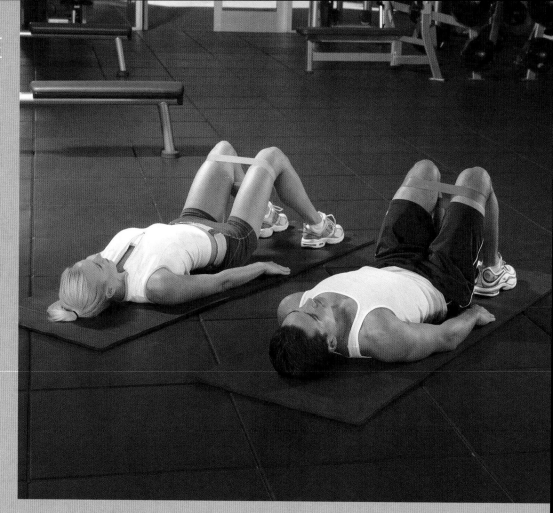

Get ready!

Surround your knees with a mini-band. Lie flat on your back, but bend your knees so that your legs resemble an upside-down V when viewed from the side. Plant your feet and keep your arms at your sides, palms down.

Go!

Slowly raise your butt off the floor until your body forms a straight line (albeit a diagonal one) from knees to shoulders. Count to one or two before slowly lowering yourself down.

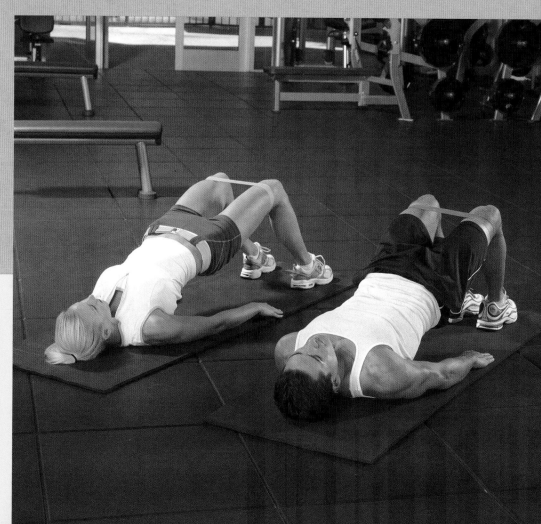

Watch out for:

Your neck coming out of alignment with your body. To help prevent this, stare at the ceiling throughout the movement.

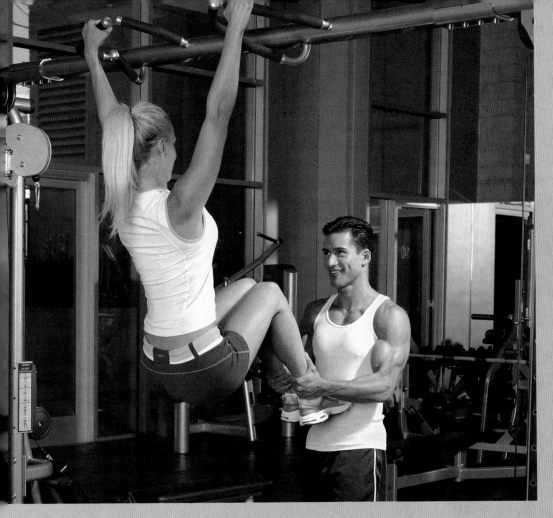

PULLUP (ASSISTED)

Great for: rock climbing, gymnastics

Get ready!

Grasp the bar overhead with an overhand grip (palms forward), so that your hands are spaced slightly wider than your shoulders. Hang freely, but bend at the waist so that your legs are extended in front of you. Your spotter should cup your feet with his or her hands. Pull down your shoulder blades.

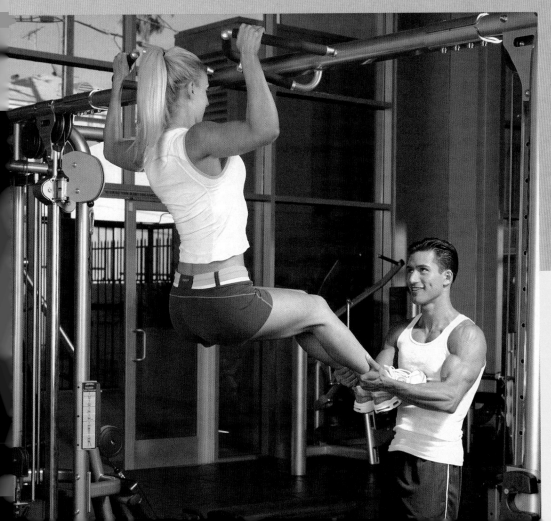

Go!

Pull your face up to the bar, squeezing your lats as your ascend. If you need assistance, press your heels into your spotter's hands. Without letting your body drop, lower yourself back to the starting position.

Tweak:

To make your core work as hard as your biceps and back, straighten your legs out in front of you, so that your body resembles the letter L when viewed from the side.

PULLDOWN

Great for:
swimming, kayaking

Get ready!

Sit down at a lat pulldown station and grab the bar above using an overhand grip, so that your hands are spaced wider than your shoulders. Keeping your head straight and back aligned, pull your shoulder blades down.

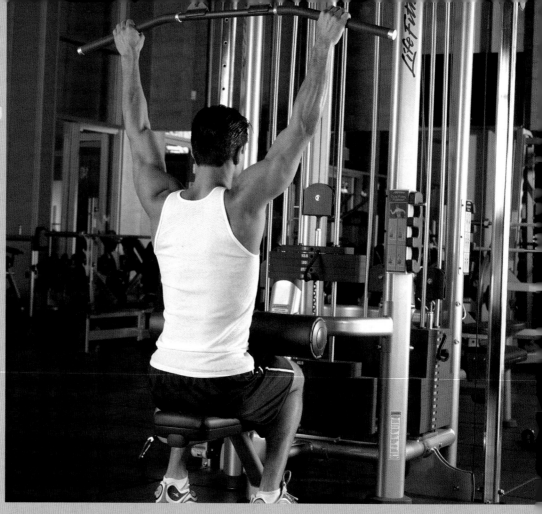

Go!

Pull the bar to your upper chest. Slowly let the bar rise back to the starting position.

Watch out for:

Pulling the bar too low on your chest, which can injure your shoulders.

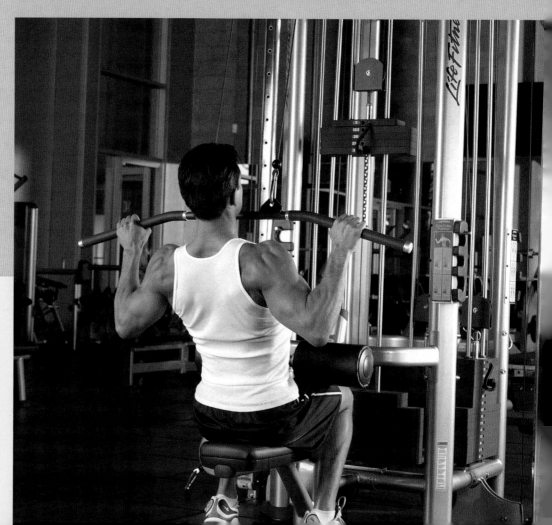

28

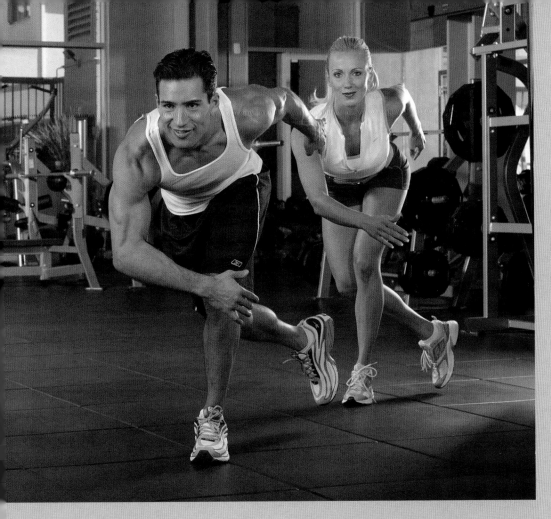

SPEED SKATING DRILL

Great for: tennis, hockey

Get ready!

Stand with your hips and knees bent and your hands on your hips.

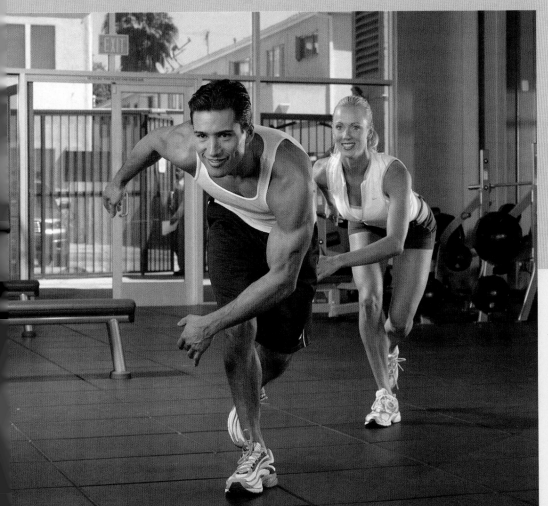

Go!

Sidestep to the right, and as soon as you've planted that foot, bring the other leg over as well, planting that foot behind the lead foot. Continue in this fashion for 10 steps before reversing the move and doing the same number of steps in the other direction.

Watch out for:

A clear path to either side. You'll be facing forward, so avoid tripping over dumbbells, weight plates, or fellow gym members.

29

SEATED DUMBBELL CURL/ SHOULDER PRESS

Great for:
lacrosse, rugby

Get ready!

Sit on a flat bench with a small back support holding a pair of dumbbells at arm's length. Your palms should be facing forward.

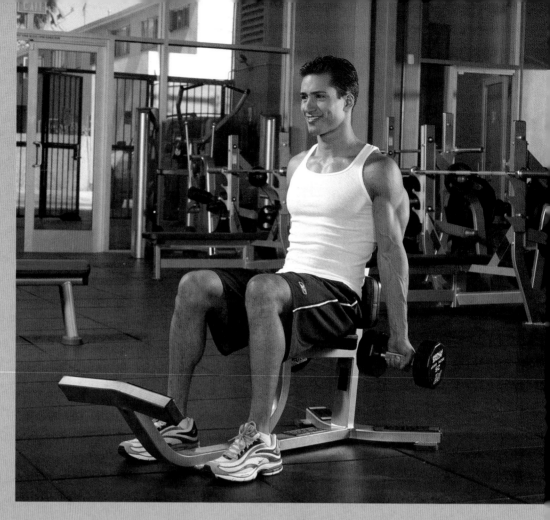

Go!

Simultaneously raise both dumbbells in a curling motion toward your shoulders. As you curl, turn your wrists so your palms are facing forward.

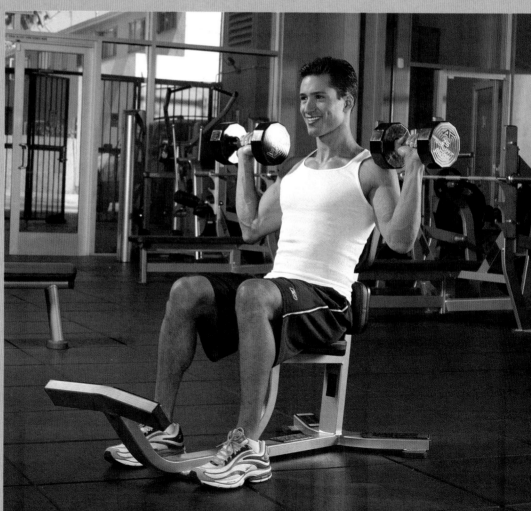

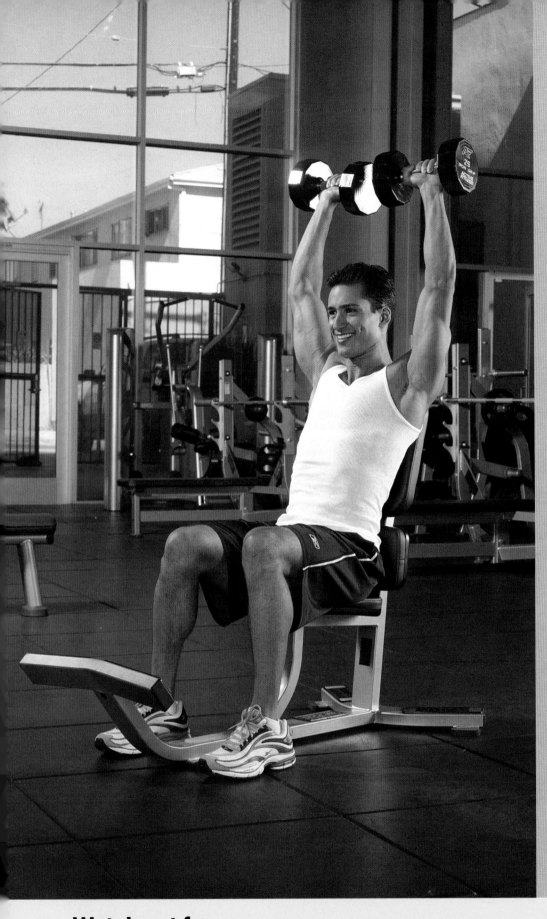

In one fluid motion, continue pressing the dumbbells overhead until your arms are fully extended. Reverse the movement, slowly and smoothly bringing the dumbbells back to your sides.

Watch out for: Excessive momentum. Don't throw the dumbbells overhead with the momentum generated by the curl. Treat the second half of the exercise—the overhead press—as a separate and distinct move.

REVERSE CRUNCH

Great for:
gymnastics, soccer

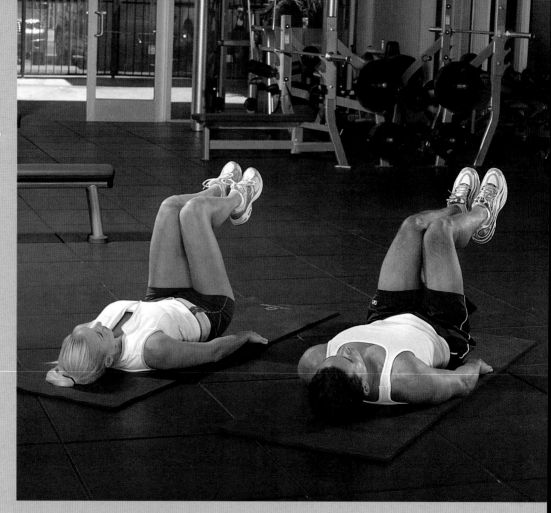

Get ready!

Lie flat on the floor, but bend your knees so that your legs form 90-degree angles when viewed from the side.

Go!

Raise your knees to your chest by pulling your hips up and in toward your torso. Lower your legs back to the starting position in a controlled motion.

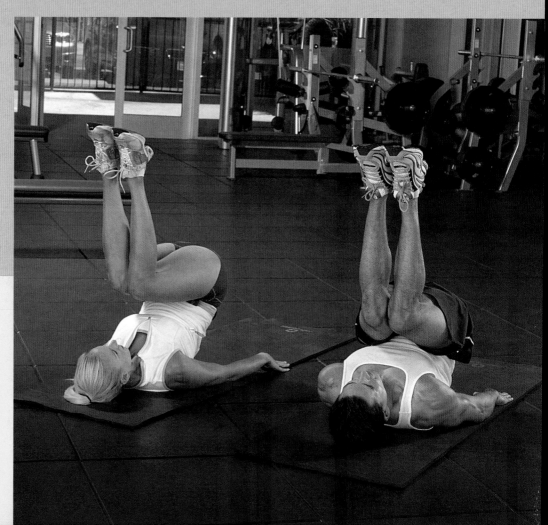

Watch out for:

Insufficient range of motion. To receive this move's full benefit, bring your hips all the way off the floor at the top of the move.

32

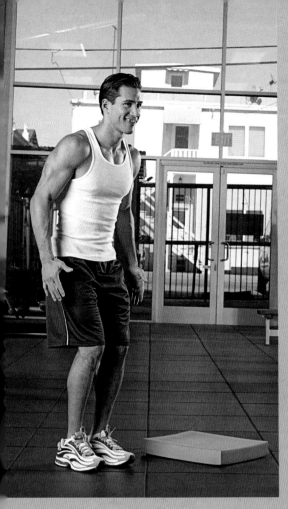
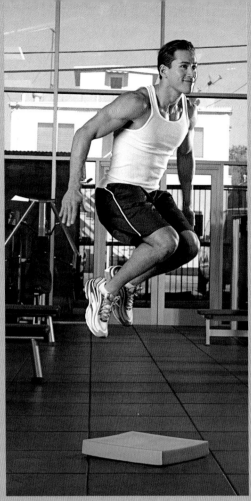

LATERAL HOPS

Great for: basketball, baseball

Get ready!

Stand to one side on a foam pad with your knees slightly bent.

Go!

Hop over to one side and then back to the starting position. Continue alternating.

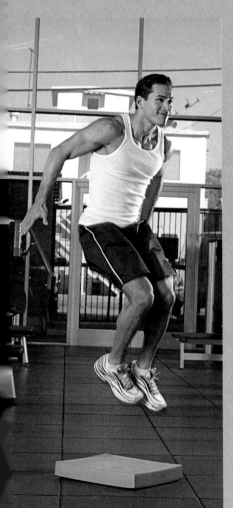
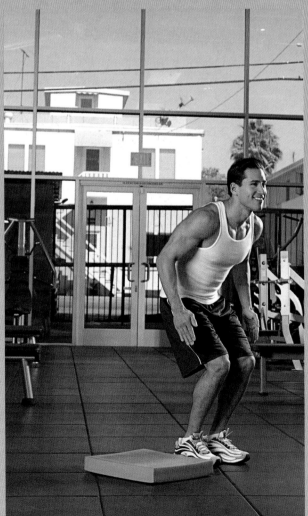

33

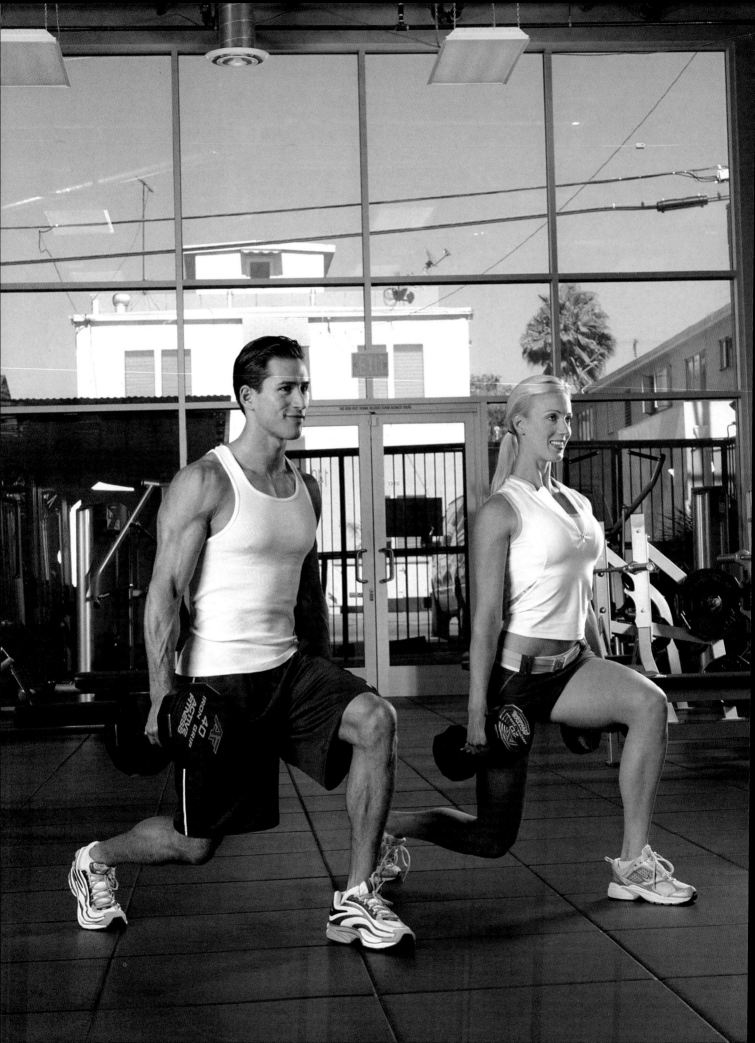

Phase I:
Workout B

Sequence	Week	Exercise	Sets[1]	Reps[2]	Rest[3]
A1	1	Dumbbell Sumo Squat	3	12–15	↓
	2	Dumbbell Sumo Squat	3	12–15	↓
	3	Dumbbell Sumo Squat	3	12–15	↓
	4	Dumbbell Sumo Squat	3	12–15	↓
A2	1	Dumbbell Alternating Chest Press	3	12–15/side	60
	2	Dumbbell Alternating Chest Press	3	12–15/side	60
	3	Dumbbell Alternating Chest Press	3	12–15/side	60
	4	Dumbbell Alternating Chest Press	3	12–15/side	60
B1	1	Lying Leg Curl	3	10–12	↓
	2	Lying Leg Curl	3	10–12	↓
	3	Lying Leg Curl	3	10–12	↓
	4	Lying Leg Curl	3	10–12	↓
B2	1	Seated Cable Row	3	12–15	60
	2	Seated Cable Row	3	12–15	60
	3	Seated Cable Row	3	12–15	60
	4	Seated Cable Row	3	12–15	60
C1	1	Reverse Fly	3	12–15	↓
	2	Reverse Fly	3	12–15	↓
	3	Reverse Fly	3	12–15	↓
	4	Reverse Fly	3	12–15	↓
C2	1	Standing Dumbbell Hammer Curl	3	12–15	60
	2	Standing Dumbbell Hammer Curl	3	12–15	60
	3	Standing Dumbbell Hammer Curl	3	12–15	60
	4	Standing Dumbbell Hammer Curl	3	12–15	60
D1	1	Superman	3	10–12/side	60
	2	Superman	3	10–12/side	60
	3	Superman	3	10–12/side	60
	4	Superman	3	10–12/side	60
E1		Perform lateral hop intervals. Do 6–8 reps of 20–30 seconds of hops, following each rep with 60–90 seconds of easy jogging in place.			

[1] Do modified supersets with each pair of exercises listed with the same number (for example, A1 and A2); that is, do the prescribed number of sets for each of the two exercises in alternating fashion before moving on to the next pairing. (For example, if the program calls for three sets, do one set of split squats followed by one set of push-ups, and then repeat twice). Rest in between each set as prescribed.

[2] The last rep you can finish with complete control and perfect form should fall within this range, so select your weight accordingly. Once you have completed all your repetitions with your current weight for two consecutive workouts, increase your poundage slightly. Five pounds for each new step is a good rule of thumb.

[3] Between supersets, measured in seconds.

DUMBBELL SUMO SQUAT

Great for:
football, volleyball

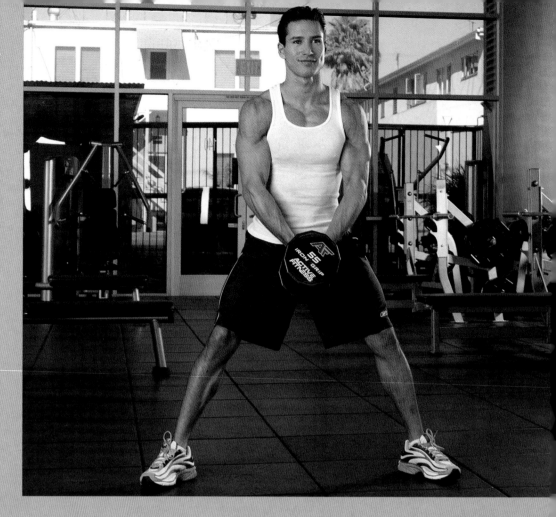

Get ready!

Stand, holding a dumbbell in front of your waist.

Go!

Bend your hips and knees to lower your torso. Descend until your thighs are parallel with the floor. Return to a standing position.

Watch out for:

Excessive upper body movement. If you're using your legs, hips, and lower back as a unit, like you're supposed to, your torso should remain stable.

36

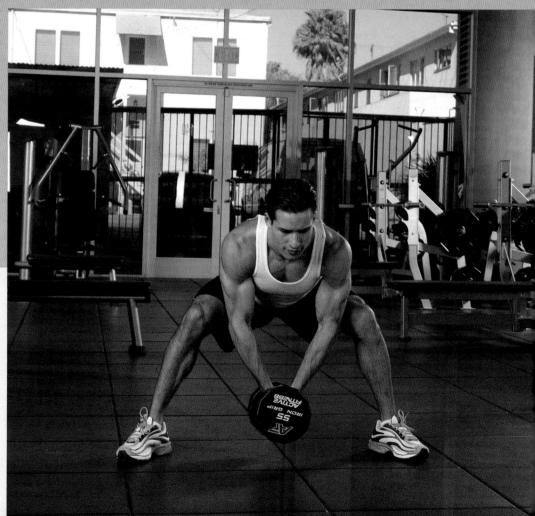

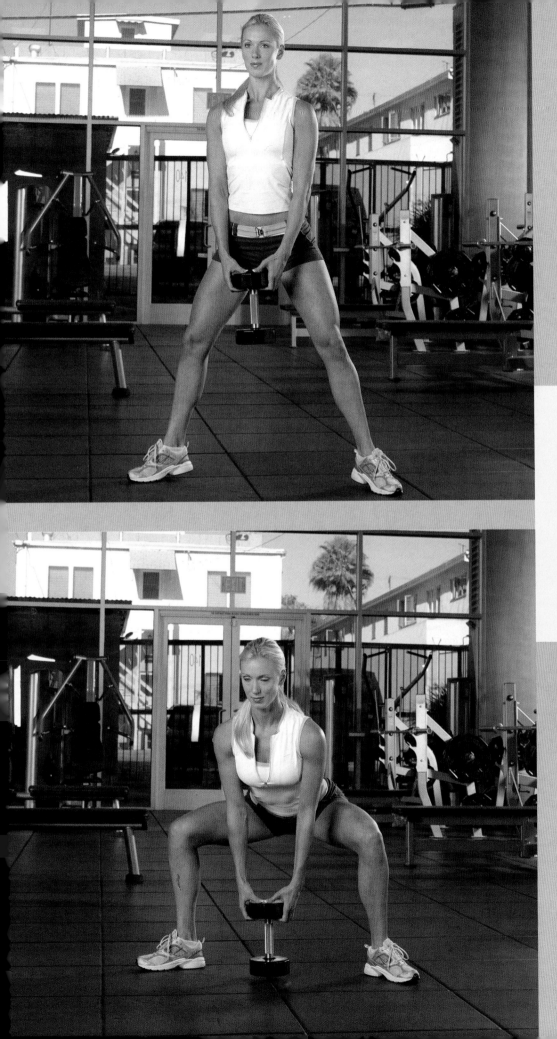

Tweak:
Women might prefer doing the plié version of this move: toes pointed out slightly wider, dumbbell held by one of the weight plates, not by the handle.

37

DUMBBELL ALTERNATING CHEST PRESS

Great for:
boxing, hockey

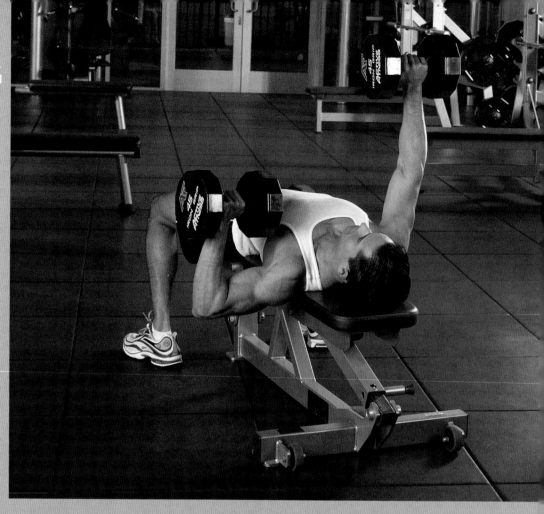

Get ready!

Lie on a flat bench looking up at the ceiling, holding dumbbells at your shoulders, palms facing up.

Go!

Holding one dumbbell motionless, press up the other until that arm reaches full extension. Repeat using the other arm, and continue in alternating fashion.

Tweak:

Push with your legs as well as your arms. Grip the ground with your toes.

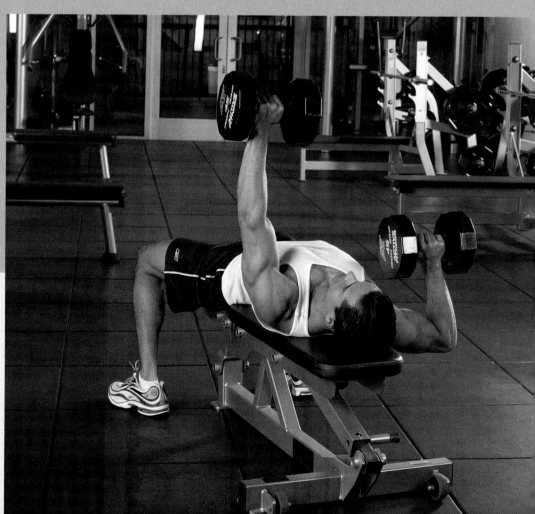

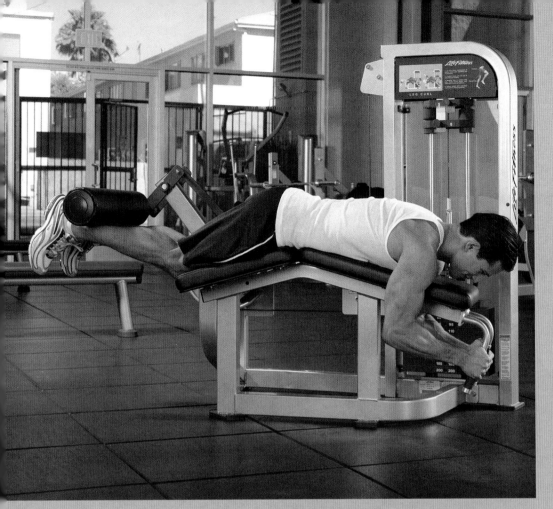

LYING LEG CURL

Great for:
swimming, soccer

Get ready!

Adjust the machine so that that roller pads fit snugly over the back of your ankles, then lie face-down. Firmly grasp the handles.

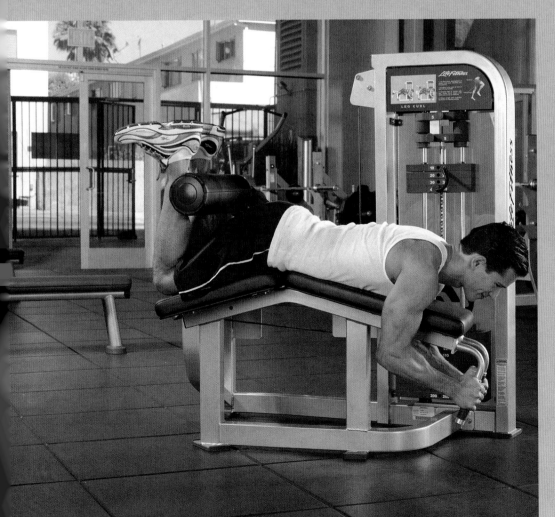

Go!

Bend your knees and flex your hamstrings to pull the roller pads up to your butt. When you can raise them no farther, stop for a one-second squeeze and return to the starting position.

SEATED CABLE ROW

Great for: rowing, tug of war

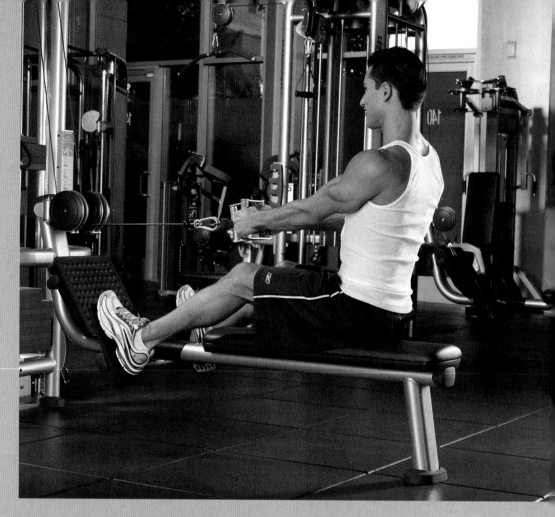

Get ready!

Attach a bar to a low cable pulley. Sit on the bench or floor and bend forward to grab the bar.

Go!

Keeping your back straight and your knees slightly flexed, pull the bar inward toward your chest, squeezing your shoulder blades together. Return to the starting position without leaning forward.

Watch out for:

Excessive momentum. Resist the weight as it pulls your arms back out in front of you on the negative half of the rep.

40

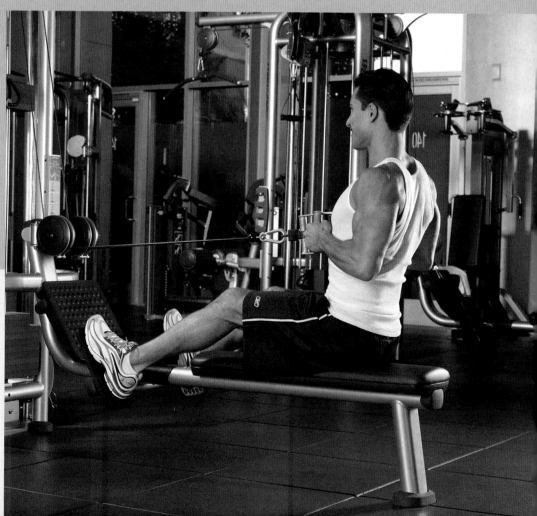

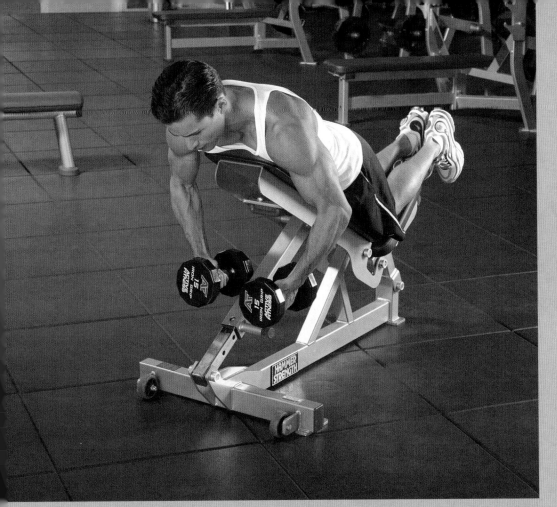

REVERSE FLY

Great for:
swimming, golf

Get ready!

Lie face-down on an incline bench— ideally the angle should be 45 degrees—with two dumbbells dangling at arm's length.

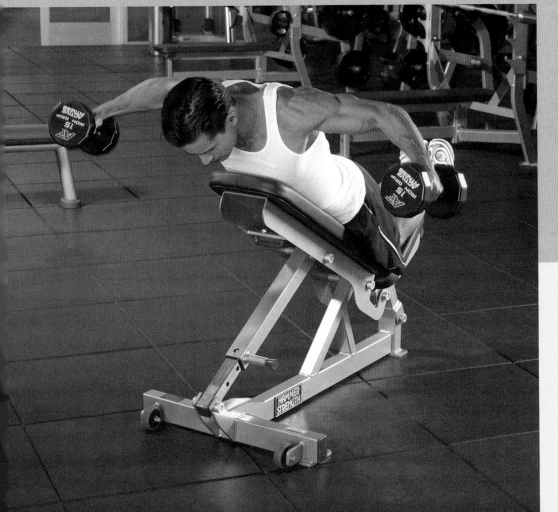

Go!

Keeping your elbows bent but your wrists straight, slowly raise your arms straight out to the sides, squeezing shoulder blades together. Return to the starting position.

Watch out for:

Looking up at yourself in the mirror. We've all done it, but it's bad. Look a few feet ahead of the bench instead. That will keep your head and spine aligned.

STANDING DUMBBELL HAMMER CURL

Great for: bowling, arm wrestling

Get ready!

Stand with your feet slightly less than shoulder-width apart. Holding a pair of dumbbells at your sides with a neutral grip, your palms facing each other.

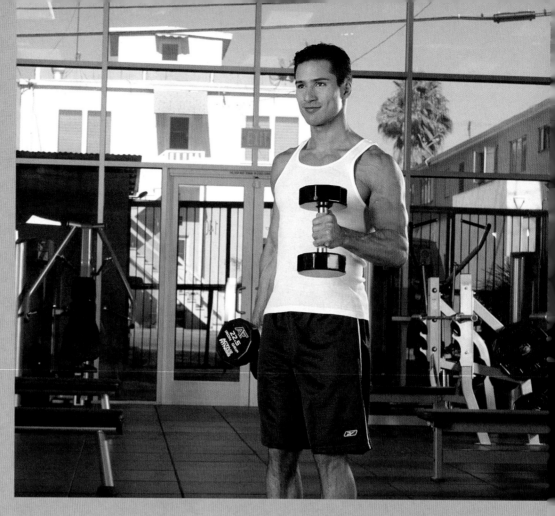

Go!

Begin raising one dumbbell up toward your shoulder in a curling motion. Do not allow your shoulder or elbow to move forward; also guard against your elbows moving out to the side. When the dumbbell is just in front of your shoulder, reverse the movement. Repeat using the other arm and continue alternating.

Watch out for:

Cheating. Keep your abs drawn in and your back straight throughout the entire set. No rocking back and forth!

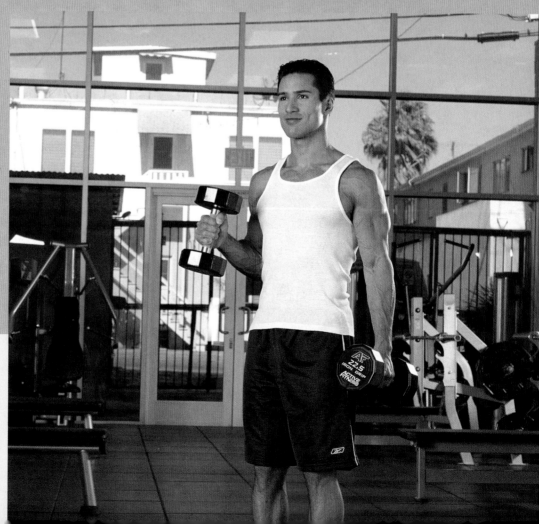

Great for: gymnastics, dance

Get ready!

Lie face-down on a mat with your arms extended in front of you, hands shoulder-width apart, and your legs extended behind you, feet together.

Go!

Time to take off! Simultaneously lift your arms and legs slightly off the ground, and hold them aloft for 10 seconds. Return to the starting position.

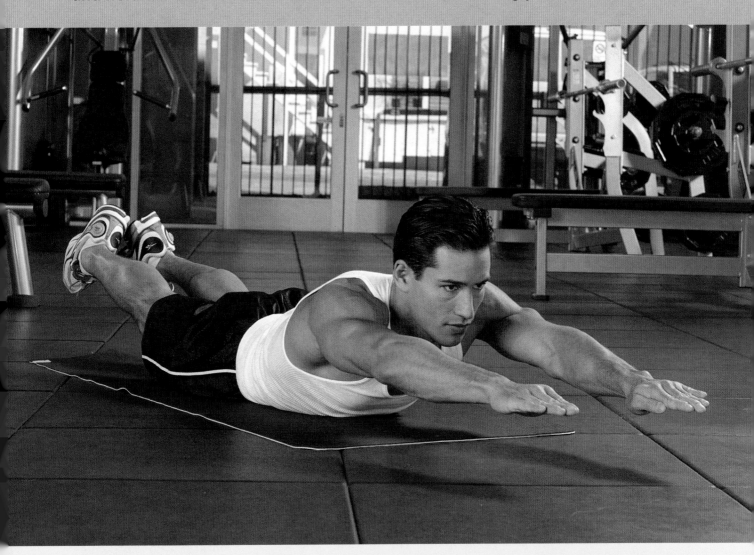

Watch out for:

The tendency to raise your head. Keep your neck in a safe alignment with your body at all times.

Phase I:
Workout C
STRIKING POWER:
MY BOXING WORKOUT

Some people play in basketball or softball leagues. I'm in a fighting league. I train to fight in "smokers," which are basically three-round amateur events. They're held at Wall Court Boxing Club, where I train. So far, I'm 7–0, with seven knockouts. Not bad, huh?

A big misconception about boxing is that it's for men only. In fact, some of the best fighters I've ever seen, pound for pound, were women. They train at my gym all the time—ladies who can throw hooks and jabs like Ali, only they don't pack quite the punch that he did because of their size. If you're a woman and you haven't tried boxing yet, I would really encourage you to give it a whirl. Men won't make fun of you; on the contrary, they'll admire you if you're already good, and want to help you if you're just starting out. You'll also complete an amazing workout, which will help lean out your body, making you look even fitter and more attractive than you already are. Plus, you'll learn self-defense while you're shaping up.

I love boxing. I used to do it almost every day, but it would be really hard on my hands, and I would wear myself out. The sport is also tough on the shoulders. Now that I box three days a week, it's great. I give my body a break, and then I hit it hard the next time out. So the three days in the boxing gym are intense, they're fun, and still frequent enough that I'm improving, not treading water—and I'm not beating up my body.

Having said that, I'm only going to ask all of you, men and women alike, to do boxing drills one day a week at first. The three gym workouts are pretty intense as it is, and we don't want you to become overtrained, especially this early in the program. Later, you'll consistently be able to hit the regular gym three times a week and a boxing gym three more times. For now, that's too much training and not enough rest.

The weight room workouts in the book will really help you in the ring as well. Especially good for boxing are the plyometrics moves in each phase. What are plyometrics? "Plyometrics activates the myostatic stretch reflex—a rubber band–like effect that enables the body to recoil with maximum power," says

Tom Seabourne, Ph.D., a professor of exercise science at Northeast Texas Community College in Mt. Pleasant, Texas. Translation: better leg work and more punching power. The intervals you perform three times a week as part of your regular workouts will help with your boxing workouts, too.

While the gym helps with your boxing, boxing in turn helps improve your gym workouts while conditioning your body. When you're dancing around the bag, you're working your legs, hips, and calves. When you're throwing hooks, jabs, and different combinations into the bag, you're working different body parts and muscle bellies. Just look at the defined back and shoulders of boxers, all from hitting that heavy bag. And ladies, think about how beautiful your shoulders are going to look in a strapless dress. As for cardiovascular training, fugheddaboutit! Nothing works out your heart like boxing does.

More and more gyms today fill entire sections and rooms with mitts, heavy bags, jump ropes, and other instruments of the sweet science. If yours doesn't, go ahead and take the plunge by joining a local boxing gym. Eventually, you'll want to anyway. That's how confident I am that you're going to love this sport.

My Boxing Workout

1) Bob-and-weave rope drill

2) Mitt drill

3) Shadow boxing drills with band resistance

4) Heavy bag training

5) Speed bag training

- Beginners should start out with 1 minute of work for each drill listed below, followed by 1 minute of recovery. Repeat each drill before moving on to the next, so that you perform 2 sets of each.
- Intermediate trainees should work up to 2 minutes of work for each drill listed below, followed by 1 minute of recovery. Repeat each drill before moving on to the next, so that you perform 2 sets of each.
- Advanced trainees should work up to 3 minutes of work for each drill listed below, followed by 1 minute of recovery. Repeat each drill before moving on to the next, so that you perform 2 sets of each.

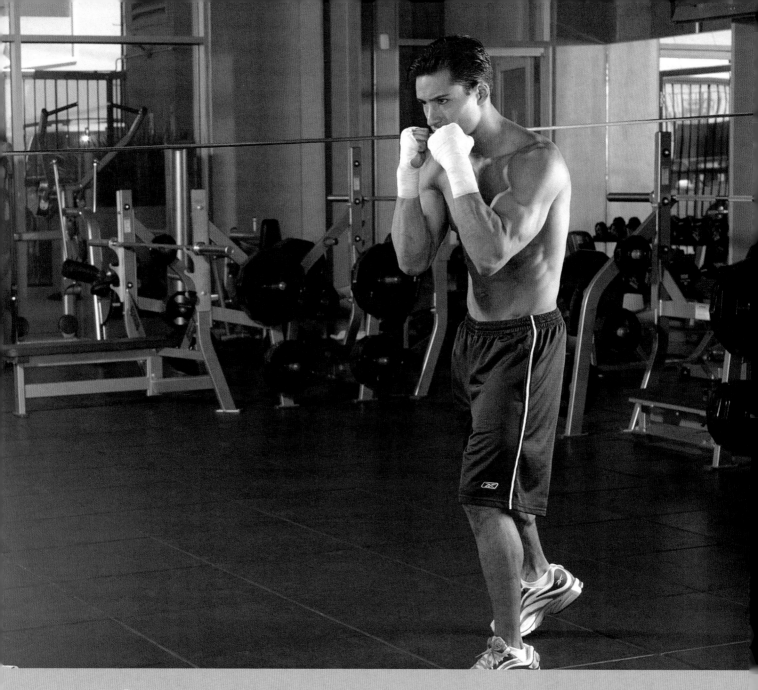

BOB-AND-WEAVE ROPE DRILL

Stretch elastic tubing in between two supports in the gym so that it lies just above shoulder height in your boxing stance. Beginning with your feet spaced shoulder-width apart and your knees and hips slightly bent, step forward and throw a jab. Imagine seeing something on the shelf in front of you. Reach forward to grab it and then bring your arm back as quickly as possible. Duck under the string, leading with your shoulder and knee, landing you on the other side of the string. Step forward, throw another jab, and then duck back under to the other side. Continue in alternating fashion.

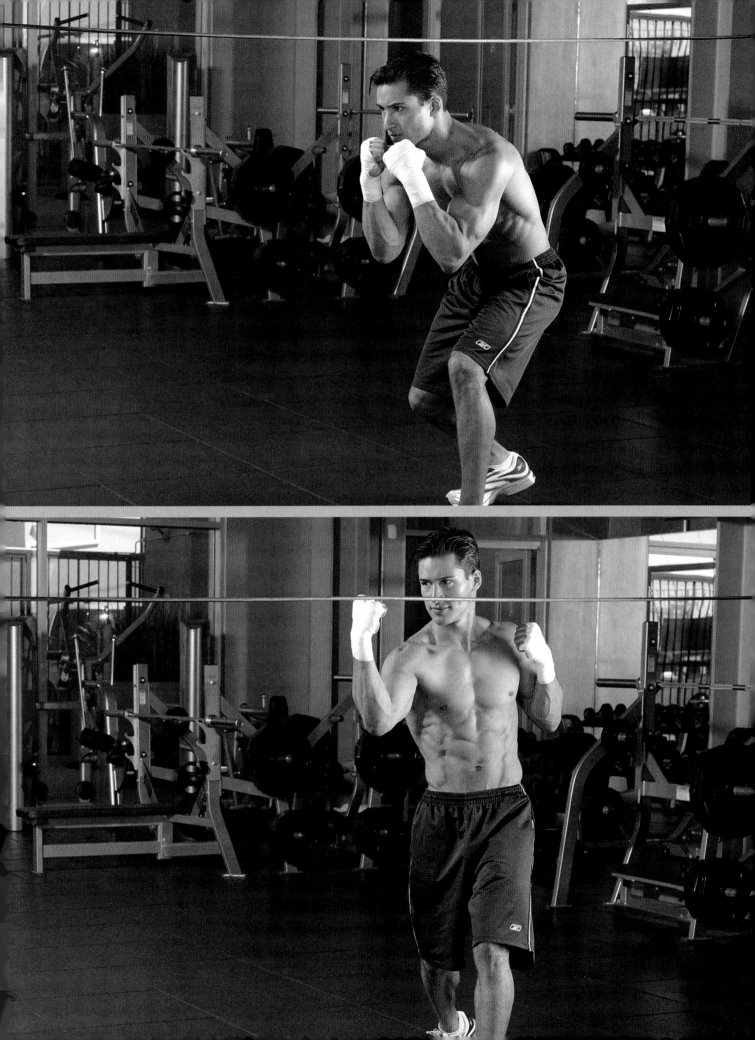

MITT DRILL

Face a partner straight on, keeping your knees bent and resting on the ball of your back foot. Keeping your abs tight, begin jabbing the mitts, alternating hands in rapid fashion. Make sure to extend each arm fully. The key is to work for speed. After a few rounds of jabs (See Bob-and-Weave Rope Drill for technique) move to hooks. Lock onto the target, begin bringing the arm you're punching with out to the side, and pivot at the hips to allow you to throw the punch forward. Rotate your wrist so that your palm faces down at full arm extension.

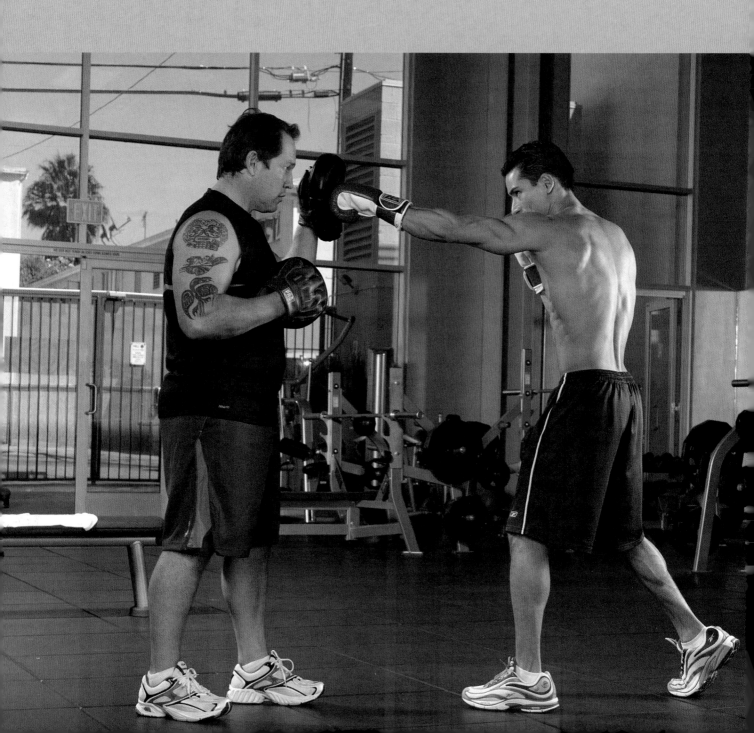

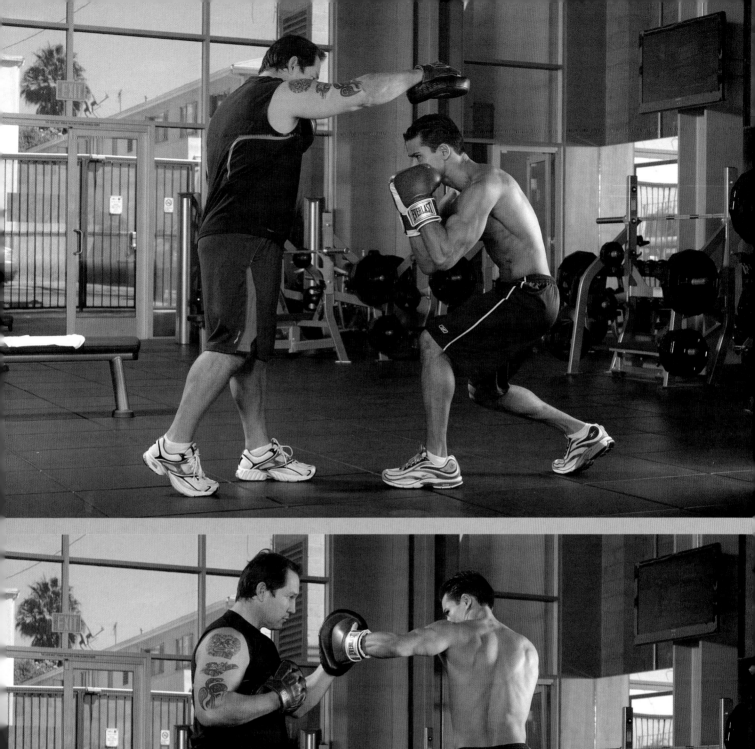
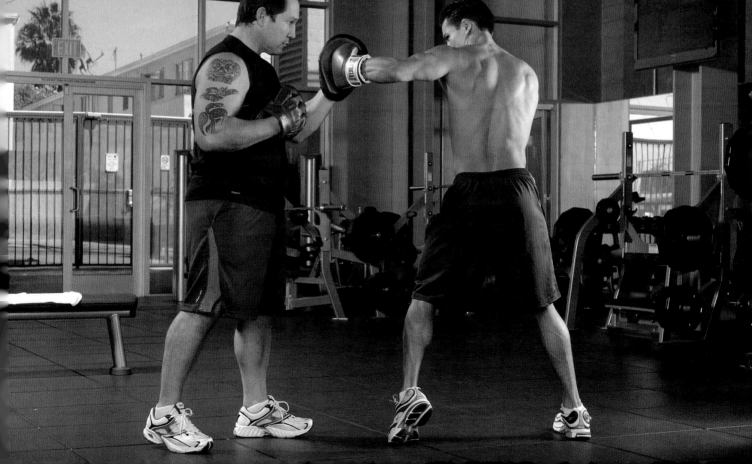

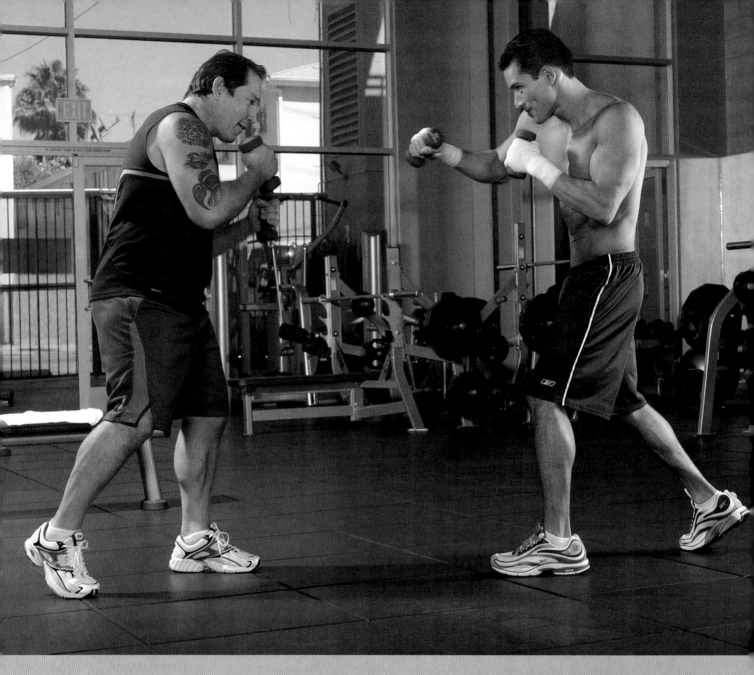

SHADOW BOXING DRILLS

Raise your hands into the ready position. With one foot in front of the other, knees bent, and abs tight, begin circling slowly, throwing jabs and hooks. Step to the side with your lead foot, bring the trailing foot behind it, and continue circling in this way. Keep your hands high, practicing to protect yourself at all times.

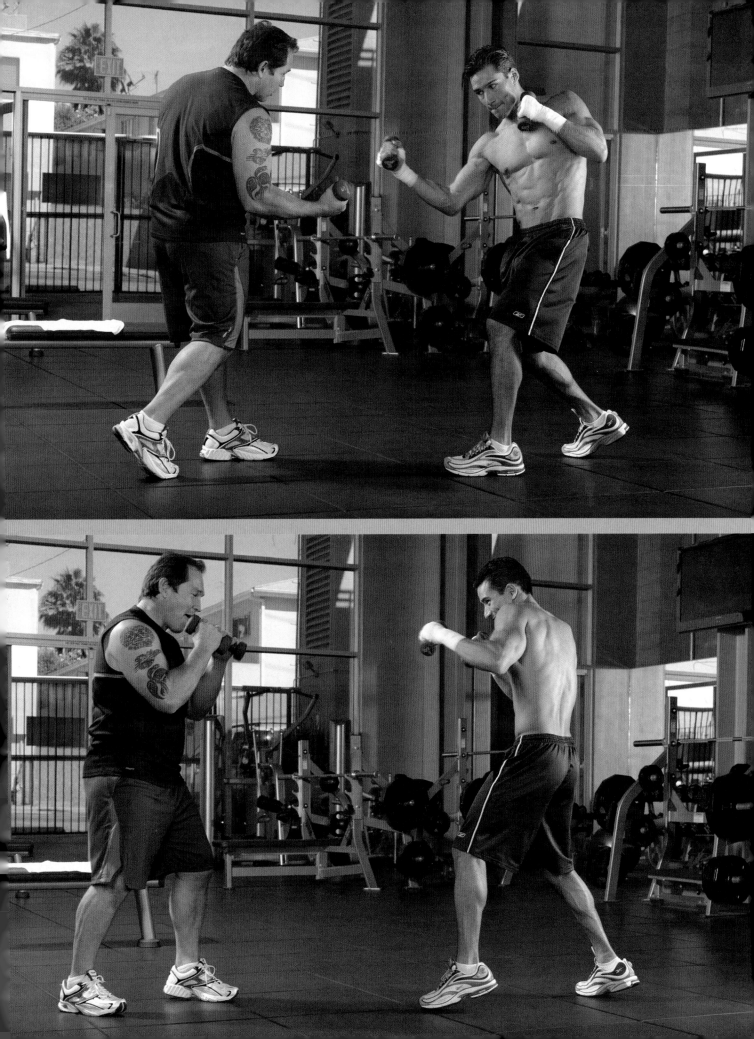

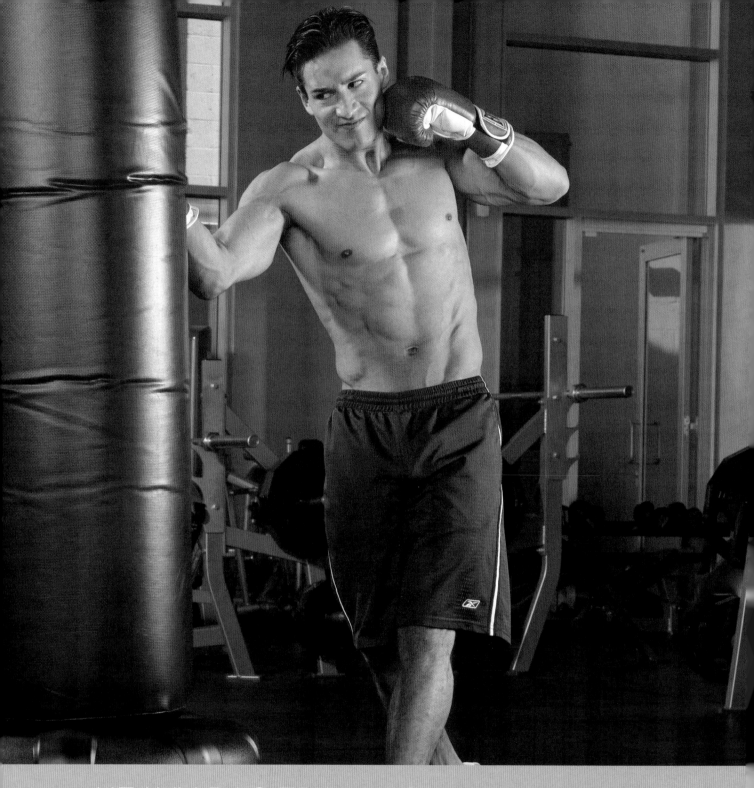

HEAVY BAG TRAINING

Strap on a pair of boxing gloves or mitts. With your knees bent and abs tight, begin leaning toward the bag by driving through your back leg and twisting your hips to generate power. Hit the bag at a point near full arm extension. Never hyperextend your joints as you strike the bag.

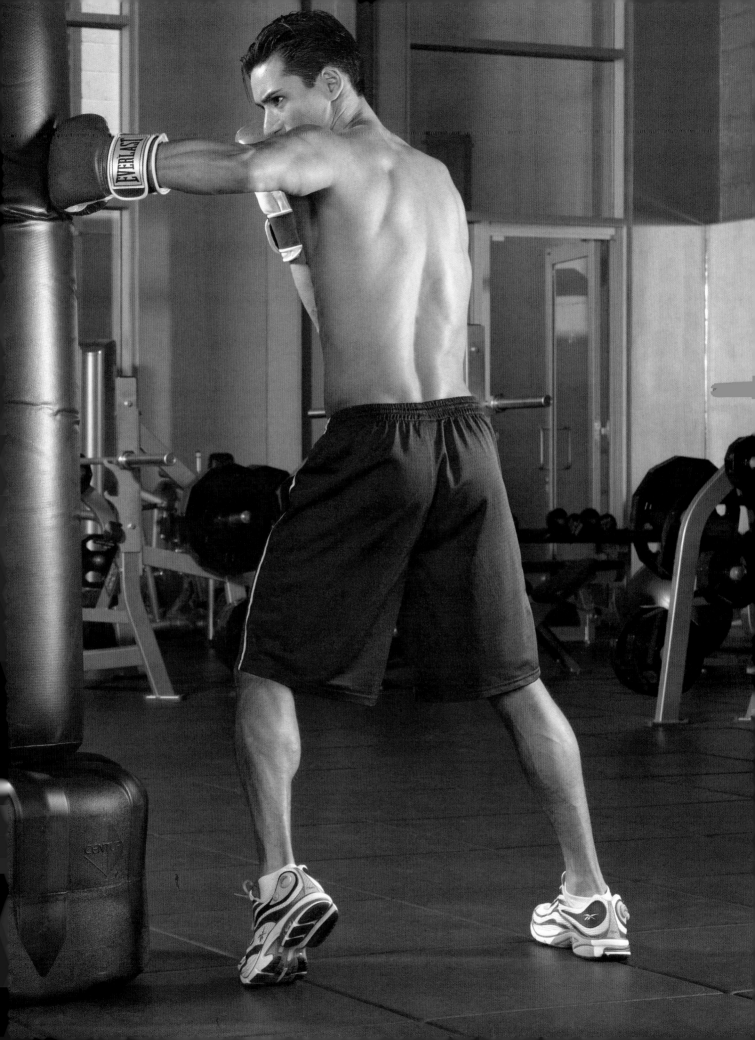

SPEED BAG TRAINING

The speed bag is all about rhythm, so keep your hands at shoulder level while maintaining small circular motions with your arms and hands. If you allow your hands to go too high or fall too low, you'll lose the tempo. After striking the bag, allow it to hit the back part of the platform, then the front part, then the back part before striking again.

I like wrapping my hands, but it's up to you. Wraps usually come with instructions, but just in case, begin by wrapping the tape around your thumb. Next, spread your fingers, and wrap the tape around your knuckles. Wrap around your wrist after that. Repeat on your other hand. At that point, dare I say it—it's a wrap!

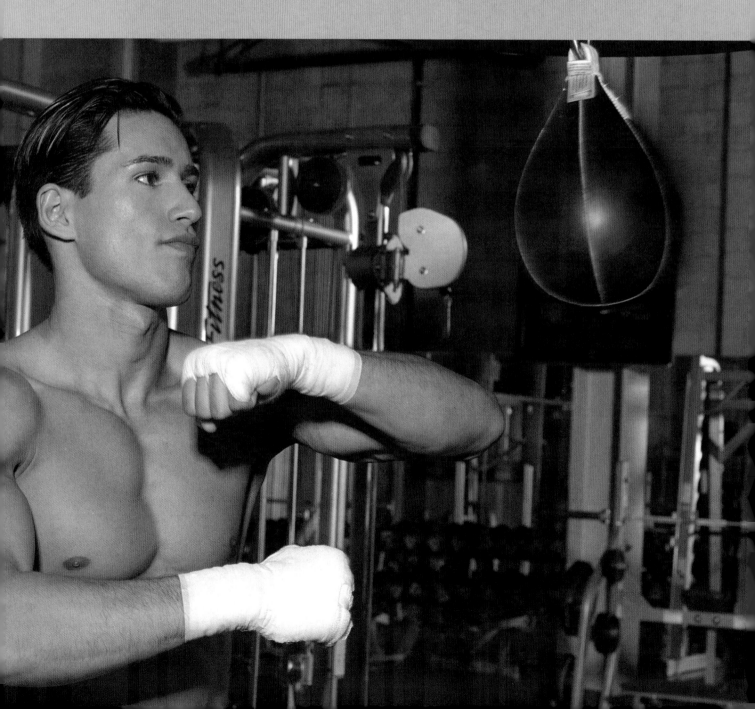

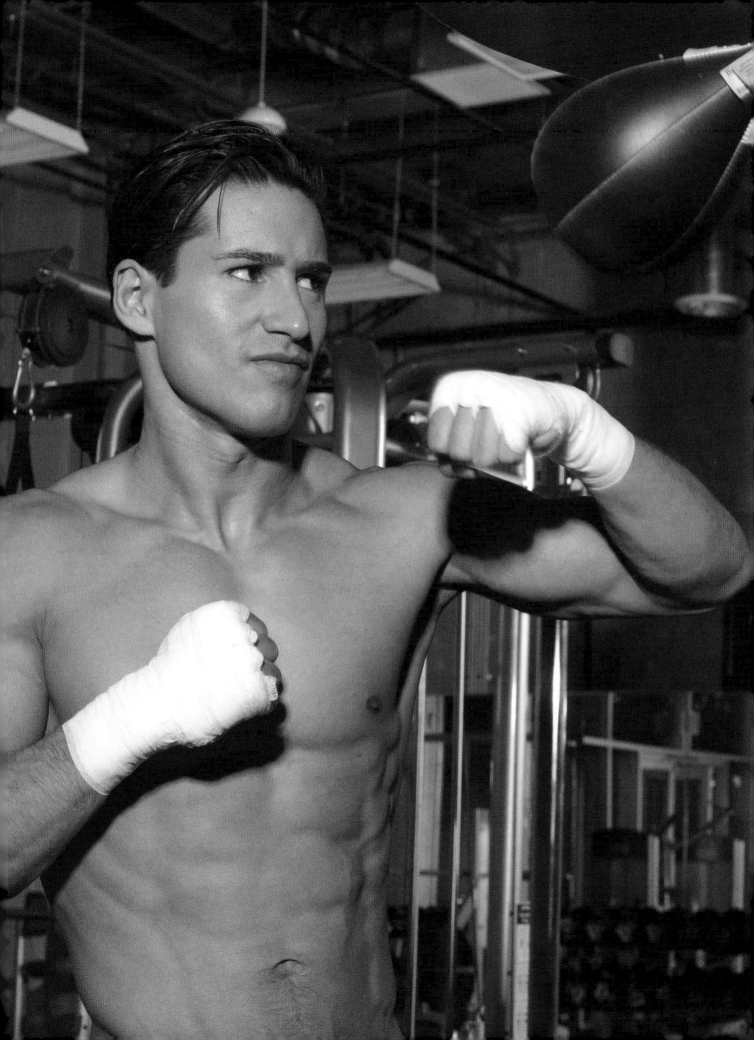

Phase I:
Workout D
HITTING THE HILLS: MY RUNNING/ BIKING WORKOUTS

I used to like to run, but ever since I bought an iPod, I *love* to run. I cue up my 80s mix play list, hit the road, and on a good day, I feel like can run forever. But I also like hiking and riding a bike, so I mix it up.

I go to the beach and run there. I climb bleachers at a local high school football stadium, run the track at UCLA, or climb those long, steep steps in Santa Monica that always set the scene for TV shows. I live in a really hilly part of the city, and one of my favorite runs is right here by my house. This hill is so steep, in fact, that even hiking at a really quick pace becomes a killer workout. When I reach the top of the hill, I feel like Rocky Balboa.

Don't think that the squats, bench presses, and other compound moves you're doing in the gym won't help you run fast, either. There's a reason Olympic sprinters are big-time gym rats sporting long cords of lean muscle: They're propelled down the track as much by their arms as by their legs.

You can also choose biking for this part of the program, or mix it up by both running and biking. I really encourage you to try both. When I first started biking, I developed my fitness by a) riding a lot and b) going out and riding with people who were one notch faster than me. Only *one* notch, though. With biking, it's very easy to jump into the deep end and find yourself in over your head (which should always be covered with a helmet, by the way—safety first). Injuries and accidents happen when you try to go faster than you can reasonably and safely go, given your experience and current fitness level.

Some tips on buying a bike: Choose one from a good local bike shop where the staff rides the way you plan to ride. If you're planning to do mostly road riding—which is best for working out, and which is what I do mostly, as opposed to off-road work—ask the guys at the shop, "Hey, what kind of rides do you do?" If they're not into road rides, find another shop. That's key, because if you're new to an area or the sport, you want the best advice on the right type of bike to buy, and help in scoping out the best local group rides. That will allow you to develop your biking skills safely while also increasing your fitness level.

When biking for fitness, try using an interval-based approach similar to what I

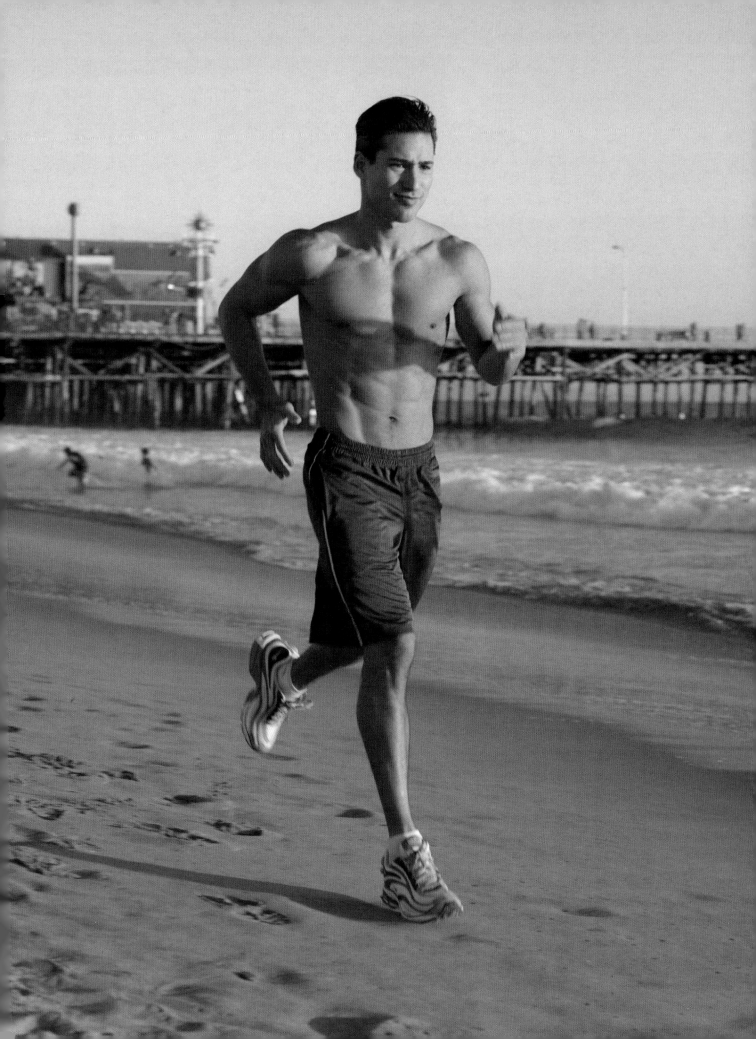

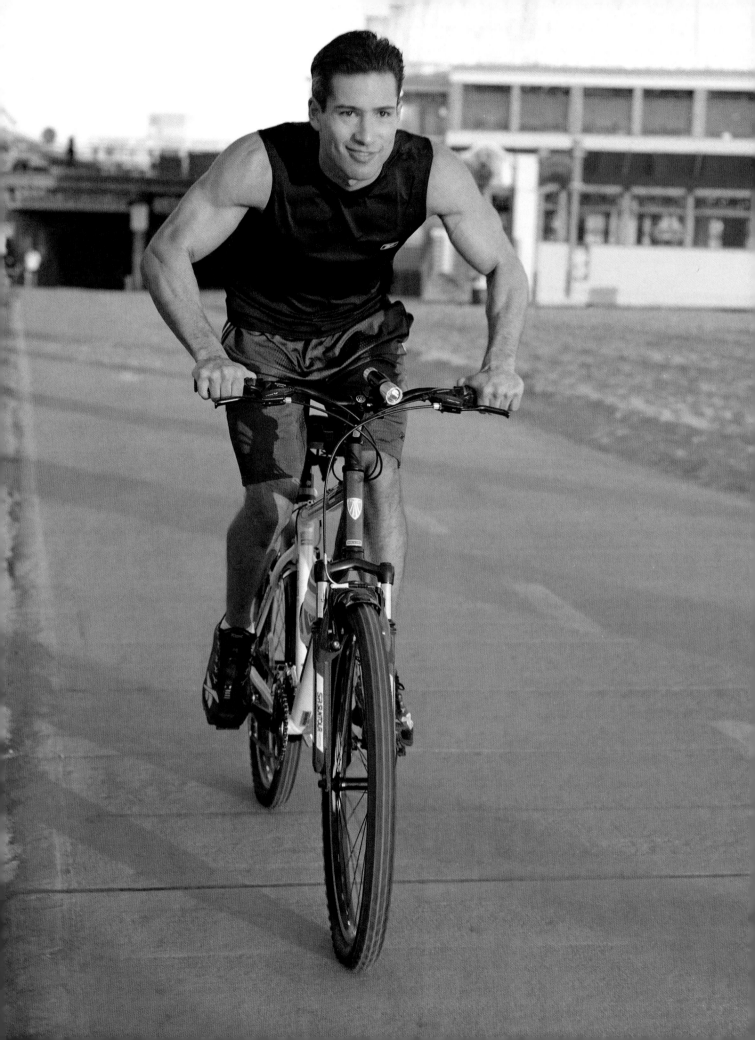

recommend for your normal cardio workouts. Think less in terms of distance and more in terms of time: Pedal vigorously for 3 minutes, back off for 3 minutes, and then continue in alternating fashion for 18 minutes. A study published in *The Journal of Strength and Conditioning Research* found that this approach improves both sprint speed and endurance. Over time, increase the length of your work intervals to 5 minutes, while keeping the less intense periods the same time; and increase the length of the overall workout up to 32 minutes. After finishing the workout portion of the ride, pedal around for another 10 to 15 minutes, just having fun. You're still burning calories even if you're not hitting it as hard as before!

My Biking Workout

1) Pedal vigorously: 3 minutes

2) Pedal casually: 3 minutes
   Continue alternating for 18 minutes total. Increase the length of your work intervals to 5 minutes, while keeping the less intense periods the same time. Increase the length of the workout up to 32 minutes.

3) Pedal around for another 10 to 15 minutes, just having fun.

10-MINUTE WORKOUT: BODY-WEIGHT CIRCUIT
FOR THOSE DAYS YOU CAN'T GET TO THE GYM

The great thing about this quickie workout is that it requires no equipment, yet hits your entire body. What that means, of course, is that it can be done in your bedroom, a hotel room, in a vacant room at the office—anywhere, anytime. If you can't make your normally planned workout that day, at least shoehorn this 10-minute blast into your day somewhere.

1) Squat thrust: up to 1 minute
   (See page 108 for exercise description.)

2) Pushup*: up to 25 reps
   (See page 24 for exercise description.)

3) Jumping jacks: up to 1 minute
   (See page 105 for exercise description.)

4) Crunch: up to 25 reps
   (Lie on the floor with your knees bent about 60 degrees, feet flat. Place your hands lightly behind your head. Curl your torso forward, lifting your shoulders slightly off the floor. Lower your torso back down.)

5) Pushup: up to 1 minute
   (See page 24 for exercise description.)
   *Place your knees on the floor if necessary
   After the first circuit, rest 2 to 4 minutes. Repeat the circuit again.
   The idea is to be able to complete 1 full minute for each work interval. Once you can accomplish the maximum number of reps and 1 full minute of work for all the moves in succession, followed by 4 minutes of rest, try decreasing the rest interval until you're able to perform all of the work followed by only 2 minutes of rest.

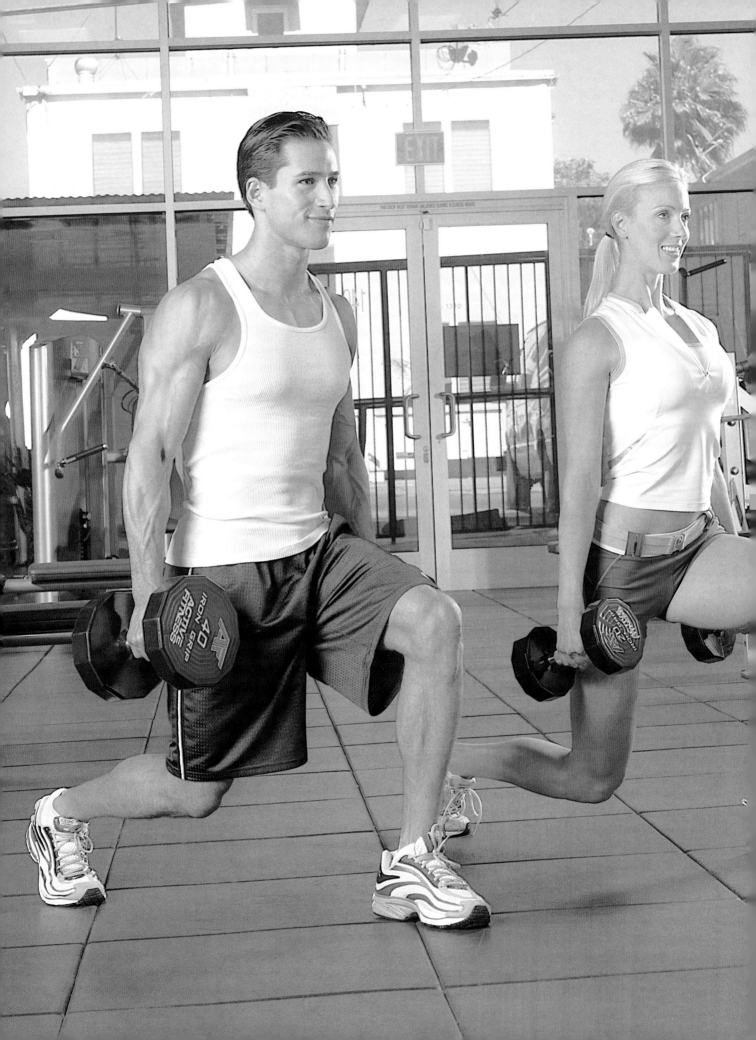

3 Meal Plans

Everyone wants a six-pack, but America is a country with an obesity problem, not an I-can't-see-my-abs problem. If half of America is on a diet, why are so many people just getting fatter?

Part of the problem is that people are relying on marketing gimmicks to help them lose weight, rather than putting down the doughnuts and picking up the dumbbells. If only someone would come out with a fat-free Oreo cookie or a magic pill, everything would be fine, right? That's always the blabber about blubber. In reality, fat-free *anything* has precious little to do with shedding pounds and getting six-pack abs. In fact, it usually has the reverse effect. In a recent experiment at Cornell University, researchers gave M&Ms to overweight subjects, telling one of the two groups they were receiving fat-free candy. Those individuals consumed nearly 50 percent more calories, on average, than their counterparts.

What's more, it doesn't take a pill, magical or otherwise, to melt away blubber. You can do it the old-fashioned way—through exercise and proper nutrition.

Proper nutrition is what this chapter is all about. As you make your way through all of my workouts, you'll encounter 21 different daily meal plans and a variety of healthy Quick & Tasty meals (designed with the help of Andrea Platzman, MS, RD), and a number of sidebars suggesting healthy items to throw on salads, supplements to take, and so on. The emphasis throughout is on what you should do, as opposed to why you should be doing it. Whenever I explain the "why," the "what" will always be there as well. The goal here is to shape you up, not prepare you to pursue an advanced degree in nutritional science. The one exception to that rule comes now, where I explain basic principles underlying my meal plans before presenting the first set of 7 (one for each day of the week).

When you follow my program, you're going to be eating like an athlete. Why so much attention to nutrition in what is, after all, a workout book? Because if you don't square away your diet, you won't be satisfied with your results, no matter what you do in the gym. Think about that: If you do every workout exactly as it's prescribed, you will still fail if you don't eat right. That goes for my book and every other workout book every written—but those authors may not have talked straight with you.

If I had to sum up my approach to nutrition and diet as they relate to working out, it would boil down to two words for men and women alike: *metabolism* and *muscle*. Metabolism is basically the number of calories your body burns on any given day. It takes calories for your heart to beat. It takes calories for digestion to occur. Even when you sleep, your body is burning calories, just to make sure you wake up when morning comes. The sum of these basic bodily processes is what's called your *resting metabolic rate*. It varies slightly depending on someone's sex, weight, and age, but for most people, this amounts to about 1,100 calories a day. Think of those as life-support calories. You can't live without 'em.

Above and beyond that, we expend more calories when we become active, whether it's walking down the street (a few calories) or sprinting as hard as we can on a treadmill (a lot of calories). The more calories you burn, the more fat you burn. Unfortunately, if you're sedentary—a couch potato who doesn't get around much—you're probably not expending much beyond that basic number (1,100 or so) that your body needs to stay alive. At the same time, let's say you're consuming 1,800 calories from your diet (which isn't that much, by the way). What happens to the extra 700 calories? Pinch your tummy and feel what happens to them.

HEY, MARIO!

Should I eat a huge meal after working out to capitalize on my super-charged metabolism?

Don't consider your workout's calorie-torching after-effects a license to splurge. Consume a protein-and-carb shake or one of the "Workout Eats" as soon as possible after training and a small, nutritious meal an hour after that. But the idea is to replenish your muscles, not gorge until you lose the metabolism-boosting benefits of your workout. Your metabolism can stay revved up for anywhere from one to eight hours, allowing you to burn an extra 50 to 200 calories.

The reverse holds true as well. If you only took in 800 calories a day—a really small number—you would be in a caloric deficit, even if you didn't engage in any physical activity. You would be burning more calories than you would be taking in. Your body would need to make up for this shortfall by finding those calories elsewhere. Eventually, it will look for fat, and burn that.

Then there's muscle. It might surprise you to learn that training actually breaks down muscle tissue. In fact, by the end of a workout, the body often finds itself in something called a *negative protein balance*. Were that condition to persist, your body would actually surrender existing muscle, not build more. That's why people talk about nutrition being 50 to 70 percent of the battle against the bulge. At least.

What you want is for your body to be recovering from a workout by rebuilding those damaged fibers. It does that by making new protein, not breaking down the existing supply. Think of muscle growth as building a brick wall. If you add four bricks (protein synthesis), but your neighbor removes six (protein breakdown), you have a smaller wall at the end of the day. But if you add six bricks, and your neighbor takes down four, you have a bigger wall. Muscle building is a constant battle between building up and tearing down.

That's how muscle growth occurs—but only if you shift that protein balance from negative to positive. Fat and carbohydrates play important roles in this process as well, but protein is the macronutrient that basically supports muscle growth. The benefits of protein don't end there, though. Researchers have found that protein slows down carbs better than even fat does. That means it also does a better job of maintaining insulin levels. In one recent study of several diets, those taking a high-protein, low-carb diet approach not only lost more body fat, but were also healthier.

Before going any further, allow me to direct a few words of wisdom to the female readers, in particular, who might worry that increasing their protein intake while lifting weights will make them look like the Incredible Hulk. Women just don't gain muscle mass as readily as men do, and eating more protein won't automatically increase their muscle growth. The difference between men and women in this regard comes down to the T factor: testosterone. So even if you're working out with great dedication and following a high-protein eating strategy, don't worry—you *will not* "bulk up." Consider it from this perspective: Think about how amazing, strong, and beautiful all the female dancers look on *Dancing with the Stars*. All of those women work out *like crazy*—more often and more intensely than anyone you know, probably. Did you ever look at one of those ladies and say, "She's too muscular?" Of course not! They all look amazing.

You *will* maintain the muscle tissue you already have, which is a very good thing. Whereas fat pretty much just sits there in the body, doing nothing but being lazy, muscle is what's called *metabolically active tissue*. That means it helps keep your fat-burning furnace stoked, which is what you want to happen.

The spacing of your meals throughout the day is also critically important. Which is why you will be eating every $2\frac{1}{2}$ to $3\frac{1}{2}$ hours, or 6 to 7 times a day. That can be a tall order for me—maybe I'm on set, on stage, in an important meeting, or in transit—but I still do my best to toe the line. Frequent feedings will provide your muscles with the nutrients they need throughout the day while keeping your metabolism elevated. It will also keep you from being hungry all the time, the way most diets make you feel. Now, you'll be eating *more* frequently, not less. Yet when you add up the total calories in these meal plans, the numbers are actually fairly low.

Compare that with what happens when you become famished, and hunger takes over. Hey, we all know the feeling, and we're all going to hit the nearest possible establishment to satisfy that craving quickly. That's the marketing genius of *fast* food. Who wants slow food, or intermediate food, when they're starving? Once you hit the drive-thru window, offers such as value meals and super-sizing for 39 cents more will seem irresistible, in part because food made from crappy carbohydrates is really cheap and accessible.

Making matters worse, reeling from hunger, you'll scarf down all that junk food so fast that your body won't have time to tell you that it's full . . . and has been for a few minutes. Your body has essentially outraced its internally generated yellow light, the one screaming, "Hey, aren't you overshooting your allotment here? Slow down!"

PROTEIN

The good kinds	**The bad kinds**
1) Seafood	**1)** Bacon
2) Beans	**2)** Sausage
3) Turkey breast	**3)** Bratwurst
4) Chicken breast	**4)** Pepperoni
5) Ostrich	**5)** Prime rib
6) Beef (100-percent grass-fed)	**6)** Fried fish
7) Eggs	**7)** Salami

Do you have any idea how many calories and how much fat you can put away at a fast food restaurant in only a few minutes? Check out some of the stats on these gut bombs:

- **Chili's Fajita Chicken Quesadillas:** 1,830 calories, 95 grams of fat (47 saturated), 151 grams of carbohydrate, 86 grams of protein
- **McDonald's Double Quarter-Pounder with Cheese and large fries:** 1,310 calories, 72 grams of fat (25 saturated), 110 grams of carbohydrate, 54 grams of protein
- **Kentucky Fried Chicken Mashed Potato Bowl with Gravy and Biscuit:** 960 calories, 46 grams of fat (12 saturated), 104 grams of carbohydrate, 31 grams of protein
- **Burger King Triple Whopper with Cheese:** 1,230 calories, 82 grams of fat (32 saturated), 52 grams of carbohydrate, 71 grams of protein
- **Hardees Monster Thick Burger:** 1,420 calories, 108 grams of fat (43 saturated), 46 grams of carbohydrate, 60 grams of protein
- **Taco Bell Express Taco Salad:** 610 calories, 32 grams of fat (10 saturated), 56 grams of carbohydrate, 17 grams of protein
- **Panda Express Orange Chicken and Fried Rice:** 950 calories, 41 grams of fat (9 saturated), 109 grams of carbohydrate, 36 grams of protein

And, last, but not least . . . gulp:

- **Macaroni Grill Primo Chicken Parmesan dinner:** 2,220 calories, 148 grams of fat (52 saturated), 126 grams of carbohydrate, 90 grams of protein

I think my abs disappeared just from typing that.

If all of us would start eating every 3 hours, every item on this America's Most-Unwanted list of gut bombs would seem much less appealing and tempting. Except maybe for the makers of fast food and cardiac stents, *everyone* would be happier.

HEY, MARIO!

I see "fat burners" in every convenience store. What are they, and can they help me lose weight?

Regardless of the marketing angle, most fat burners are slightly different variations on a formulation designed to rev your nervous system for short periods of time. That's not a particularly bad thing, per se, but it isn't for everyone, and the ingredients aren't always combined wisely or even safely. Most important, fat-burning pills burn trivial amounts of fat compared with working out and eating right. **Save your money.**

10 DIETARY MISTAKES TO AVOID

1) Not eating enough protein, especially early in the day. The government's recommendation for protein—a measly 0.4 grams per pound of body weight—is barely half of what you need to build muscle, which in turn will help you burn fat. This applies to women as well: You need protein!

2) Skipping breakfast. I don't mean grabbing a soda or eating a quick doughnut; I mean consuming whole foods such as oatmeal, eggs, fruit, milk, and yogurt. Your brain and body both need these nutrients to function.

3) Skipping other meals because you didn't think ahead. Maybe you're in meetings all day and haven't eaten for six hours. When you finally do, you choose badly because you're friggin' starved. What's more, you eat too quickly when you're famished, outracing your body's "fullness" signal. Instead, aim to eat every three hours.

4) Eating carbs only. A plain bagel alone, or with orange juice, is one of the worst breakfasts you can eat. Dreadful. Your blood sugar will light up like fireworks on the Fourth of July. This stimulates the release of the hormone insulin, which signals your body to stop burning and start storing fat. It also triggers hunger, making you reach for something else that will skyrocket your blood sugar again. Better to start your day off with eggs (protein), turkey bacon (fat), and a side of fruit (healthier carbs).

5) Thinking in terms of "snacks" packaged in boxes and bags. Stop planning your meals around snacks. Just plan frequent meals. When you do the "s" thing, you're not saving yourself calories from a meal. Oftentimes you're upping your calories.

6) Consuming cheap, crappy carbs. Non-diet soda, potato chips, cookies, popcorn, and white bread have made America fat. The empty calories are bad enough, but the real damage comes from the havoc these wreak on your blood sugar.

7) Falling for the fat-free gimmick. Just because some box of crap you bought at the store says "fat free" doesn't mean you can eat twice as much of it without ballooning your belly. You'll still be consuming a bunch of calories. What's worse, the phrase *non-fat* is usually code for—you guessed it—more sugar.

8) Not "fishing" for healthy protein. Generally speaking, plant fats are healthier than animal fats. But the fats in fish are an exception, especially those from darker fleshed ones like salmon. The omega 3 fatty acids they contain are just what the doctor ordered to keep your ticker ticking. (The U.S. government doesn't provide RDAs for omega 3s, but they should.) In the meantime, substitute fish for another animal protein several times a week and supplement with omega 3s for good measure.

9) Not drinking enough water. Your factory-installed thirst mechanism is a lemon. By the time you crave water, you're already dehydrated. That can short-circuit today's workout and eventually wreck your health, which is a shame, since all you have to do is turn on a friggin' faucet. Drink a minimum of 12 6-ounce glasses of non-caffeinated fluids per day, plus an additional 6 ounces for every 15 minutes of training.

10) Shopping in the center aisles of the supermarket. Not everything in the center aisles of your local supermarket is junk—hey, canned tuna is useful—but the vast majority of what you'll find there has been pumped full of chemicals and processed beyond belief. Unless you need a greeting card, a magazine, or a can of shaving cream, stay on the store's periphery, where all the fresh stuff lies.

Along with the timing of your meals, the *composition* of your meals is hugely important. Mix up your meals like I mix up my training, combining the three major macronutrients—protein, carbs, and fat—in the same sitting. Eating nothing but carbohydrate at one time is a blood-sugar disaster, because glucose floods your bloodstream suddenly and in large quantities. We're talking tidal wave here. The faster all that sugar arrives, the more insulin the pancreas releases. The organ basically panics, desperately attempting to shuttle that glucose from your bloodstream, where it does damage, and into your cells, where it can be used for its intended purpose—energy. The end result of huge insulin spikes from major glucose loads: you, only fatter. Instead, you want a little bit of carbohydrate, a little bit of protein, a little bit of fat, mixed together, to prevent those sugar surges.

There is one exception, and it applies only to readers of this book looking to increase their muscle mass significantly-—which means you guys, for the most part. There is one time—and one time only—when I would encourage you to unleash a bit of an insulin surge: immediately after completing one of the three weekly gym workouts. For those individuals, at that time of day, a post-workout insulin spike can increase the uptake of glucose and amino acids. Immediately after a hard workout, your body can store twice as many carbs twice as fast as it can at other times. That's why it's good to drink a shake with whey protein, branched-chain amino acids, and even carbohydrates after you finish your last rep that day.

But that's the lone exception to a key principle of healthy eating: *Do not spike your blood sugar.*

The way you mix meals should shift as the day unfolds. Breakfast is a good meal for consuming carbohydrates, especially fruit. As you move from morning into the afternoon, reduce your carbs. As you move from the afternoon into the evening, reduce that number even more. The carbs consumed later in the day should come from broccoli, cauliflower, spinach, zucchini, and other low-sugar, high-fiber vegetables. Because your body becomes less adept at handling carbohydrates as the day unfolds, those consumed later are more likely to be stored as fat.

Another tip: Become a little less concerned about fat and little more concerned about sugar and flour, if you're not already. Some fats, such as the trans fats found in cookies and other baked goods, are associated with cardiovascular disease, and should be avoided like the heart attacks they help cause. Pretty much anything battered and deep-fried spells bad news as well. Having said that, many types of fat are good for you when consumed in appropriate amounts. Plants are the best source for these beneficial fats, which include olive oil and canola oil. Avocados are one of the healthiest foods known to man, and they're loaded with (heart-healthy monounsaturated) fat. Ditto nuts and seeds. Even saturated fat, which mostly comes from animals and is solid at room temperature, may not be quite the dietary boogey-man that it's been portrayed to be for decades. When you restrict your intake of sugar and crappy carbs, the body is more likely to treat saturated fats as fuel to be burned, rather than as baggage to be stored.

As a general rule, low-fat diets don't work because they make you feel hungry all the time. An empty feeling in the pit of your gut becomes your constant companion. Fun, huh? That's because fat helps satiate you. So when you decrease your fat intake, you don't receive messages from the hormones that normally send off the "Hey, I'm full!" signals. Protein, on the other hand, encourages those hormones to send off fullness signals, thereby decreasing hunger.

HEY, MARIO!
Besides water, are there other beverages I should drink every day?

That one's easy. The closest thing we have to a fountain of youth is a steaming-hot cup of green tea (but keep in mind, green tea does contain caffeine). In a recent study, University of Minnesota scientists found that drinking just one cup a day slices your colon cancer risk in half. Better yet, drink two, three, or five cups a day. According to *Journal of the American Medical Association,* five cups are good for a 22-percent reduction in heart disease risk.

Taste is yet another reason not to eliminate all the fat from your diet. Simply put, fat makes a lot of foods taste good. Heck, one of my favorite foods ever is taking the melted cheese from the nachos at the movie theater and pouring it over the popcorn! (I don't recommend that, by the way.) The cycle goes like this: You're consuming all these really lousy-tasting foods because everything in your diet has to be "fat-free," so you're hungry all the time, and you end up breaking down and eating bad food. Fat also slows down carbohydrate digestion, so when you consume low-fat, high-carb foods—especially the faster-burning carbs we've already talked about—your body's insulin secretion will shoot through the roof.

I'm not telling you to feast on red meat every night. For your sake, lean poultry and fish should find themselves on the end of your fork more frequently than beef. What I am telling you is that enjoying a nice steak now and then won't kill you. On the contrary: When Danish researchers tracked the dietary habits of more than 42,000 men and women for five years, they discovered that the meat eaters had the smallest increases in belt size. Again, the fat in meat doesn't make you fat; it makes you full. So you stop eating. That's why I firmly believe that if you "drive through" at a fast-food restaurant, the saturated fat in that burger patty isn't your biggest concern. Worry more about the boatload of simple sugars that will flood your bloodstream from that belly-buster soda, those up-sized fries, and that refined-flour-and-high-fructose-corn-syrup-containing hamburger bun.

Diabetes is now an epidemic. Raging blood sugar, and the high levels of insulin secreted to control it, are directly related to heart disease. (My grandmother suffers from the disease, so I've seen firsthand the devastation it causes.) New research also shows that the consumption of large amounts of sugar and refined grains is significantly related to increased risk of pancreatic, esophageal, and kidney cancers. Just as frightening is what sugar can do to your brain. In a recent study, researchers found that people who drink two and a half cans of soda daily are three times more likely to be depressed and anxious compared to those who drink less. And over time, chronically elevated blood sugar levels can permanently damage brain neurons, leading to dementia and Alzheimer's.

In contrast, if there is a nutritional magic bullet for staying healthy and shedding weight, it's something decidedly unglamorous and sexy: fiber. One awesome thing fiber does is fill you up, crowding out calories that will never bulge your belt as a result. What's more, fiber takes longer to digest than other nutrients, so that feeling of fullness will linger for a good long while. Most important, fiber slows down carbohydrate digestion, preventing blood sugar spikes, insulin surges, and the resulting blood sugar crashes. Who wants to spend their day riding an energy rollercoaster?

Fiber sounds like it should be worth its weight in gold, right? So where can this amazing nutrient be found? You don't have to look hard—fruits, vegetables,

FATS

The good kinds

1) Wild salmon

2) Olive oil

3) Walnuts

4) Canola oil

5) Flaxseed/oil

6) Cod liver oil

7) Almonds

The bad kinds

1) Shortening

2) Butter

3) Margarine

4) Hydrogenated oil

5) Corn oil

6) Fried foods

7) Cream

and whole grains are all rich sources. In other words, the foods I've been encouraging you to eat all along! A day shouldn't go by without you consuming at least 30 grams of fiber. Take a supplement such as BeneFiber if that's what it takes to get your fill.

Fruits, vegetables, and whole grains are all carbohydrate foods, so this isn't a low-carb approach. I like to think of it as a *selective-carb* approach. Most people crave carbs, so when you reduce them dramatically, changes in brain chemicals such as serotonin make you feel crappy. What's more, you're going to be working out now, so you need healthy carbs to fuel those efforts.

"Healthy carbs" is the operative phrase here.

You see, eating better isn't rocket science. It mostly boils down to turning bad habits into good ones. Healthy habits include becoming organized enough to make your food, like packing your lunch in the morning. Changing only a few bad habits can keep so many other bad habits at bay. Nor does eating better make you a robot. I don't subject you to this in the meal plans, but I put lime and hot sauce on everything I eat. Maybe it's a Latin thing—who knows? All I know is it frustrates my friends when they are cooking. They're like, "I don't know why I even bother to cook because you put lime and hot sauce on everything! It all tastes the same." As I tell them, "It *enhances* the flavor of everything you're preparing!"

Stimulate your metabolism by eating as well as by exercising. You don't even need to cut out calories much to burn fat—just eat really clean, wholesome foods. The better you eat, and sometimes the more you eat, the more you're fueling your metabolism. The more cardio you do, the more you're fueling your

CARBS

The good kinds

1) Quinoa

2) Beans (black, kidney, red, pinto, etc)

3) All vegetables

4) All fruits

5) Oatmeal

6) Barley

7) Buckwheat

The bad kinds

1) White bread

2) High-fructose corn syrup

3) Rice cakes

4) Ready-to-eat cereals with fewer than 3 grams of fiber per serving

5) Sugar

6) White flour

7) French fries

metabolism. The more muscle you sprout, the more you're fueling your metabolism. It's all part of a cycle that helps speed up the process of reducing body-fat stores when you're already doing the hard work at the gym.

A final word: Jot down everything you eat or drink all day in a journal. Do it for a week or two, or maybe even a full month. Recording is probably the single best thing you can do to give yourself some feedback and get a handle on what's entering your mouth. From there you can begin to decrease or even phase out problem foods. Maintaining a food log may sound like a nuisance, and it might be at first, but I find myself scribbling down notes all the time now. Soon you'll be checking your log more frequently than the morning box scores or stock quotes. The protein, fat, and carbohydrate grams you're putting in your body are more important, anyway. This information has a direct bearing on the most important statistical result of all: your lifespan.

To craft the specific meal plans, I enlisted the help of Jim Stoppani, PhD, one of the brightest minds working in the fitness field today. Dr. Stoppani received his doctorate in exercise physiology from the University of Connecticut in 2000. Following graduation, he served as postdoctoral research fellow in the Department of Cellular and Molecular Physiology at Yale University School of Medicine, where he investigated the effects of exercise and diet on gene regulation in skeletal muscle. He knows his stuff.

To increase muscular endurance during Phase I, your body will require ample amounts of healthy carbohydrates. Your body will rely heavily on this fuel source during workouts. On days when you're *not* working out, here's what your body needs:

- Anywhere from 11 to 13 calories per pound of body weight. (I weigh 175 pounds, so that's 1,900 to 2,300 calories for me.)
- Approximately 1.5 grams of carbs per pound of body weight. (That's 260 grams of carbs for me.)
- About 1 gram of protein per pound of body weight. (That's 175 grams of protein for me.)
- Fewer than 0.5 grams of fat per pound of body weight (That's fewer than 85 grams for me.)

HEY, MARIO!

What's a quick tip for helping me gain a few extra pounds of muscle over the next month?

Before going to bed at night, eat a small meal with a protein-to-carb ratio of 2:1 or even 3:1. Example: 1 cup of cottage cheese with a handful of red grapes and raw nuts, such as walnuts or pecans. Night is both the most important time for growth and the longest time you're without calories, so if you want to maximize the benefits of your weight training, fortify your body before falling asleep.

Now do your math:

11–13 calories × (your weight) = calories per day
1.5 grams of carbs × (your weight) = carboyhdrates per day
1 gram of protein × (your weight) = protein per day
<.5 gram of fat × (your weight) = fat per day

On those days when you do work out, here's what your body needs:

- About 14 calories per pound of body weight.
  (I weigh 175 pounds, so that's 2,450 calories.)
- A little more than 1.5 grams of carbs per pound of body weight.
  (That's around 300 grams of carbohydrates.)
- A little more than 1 gram of protein per pound of body weight.
  (That's around 200 grams of protein for me.)
- Fewer than 0.5 grams of fat per pound of body weight.
  (That's fewer than 85 grams for me.)

Now do your math for your workout days:

14 calories × (your weight) = calories per day
>1.5 grams of carbs × (your weight) = carbohydrates per day
>1 grams of protein × (your weight) = protein per day
<0.5 grams of fat × (your weight) = fat per day

Follow those guidelines, and you'll have ample nutrients to recover from previous workouts and prepare for the next one, while still allowing you to get lean.

Dieting may seem like a chore that requires you to eat like a bird, but here we show you how to enjoy tasty food while still slimming down and toning up. And if you think sticking to this healthy eating plan means painstakingly preparing every meal by hand—and then carting around meals in plastic containers while everyone heads off for a nice lunch—relax. In fact, we provide several sample meals you can order at some of the more popular national chain food joints. These are the healthier alternatives to the gut bombs we mentioned before. Yes, even McDonald's is included.

These sample daily meal plans are just that, samples. They're also completely modular, so don't be afraid to mix and match. If you really like one of our sample lunches, feel free to have it on any day you prefer. If you can't make it to Wendy's on the day we recommend, any of the other healthy fast food meals

5 REASONS TO KEEP A FOOD JOURNAL

1) You won't realize what you're eating until you put it down on paper. Oh, I reach into so-and-so's desk and grab three handfuls of M&Ms! Oh, I get hungry every afternoon come 4 o'clock. I've never noticed that before! Wow, this candy bar has 250 calories, or, this jelly doughnut has 500 calories. Yikes.

2) The truth hurts. You'll automatically start cleaning up your diet just because you don't want to see some of the crap you're writing down. When it comes to food, ignorance isn't bliss.

3) You can make last-minute modifications. Seven o'clock rolls around. You scan your log and realize you haven't eaten enough vegetables today. Never fear. There's still time to add broccoli or another fibrous carb to your dinner.

4) Bad patterns emerge clearly from the food fog. Like not eating enough during the day. A lot of women I know say they're fine through the day, only to be starving at night. So they eat junk as soon as they reach home and continue until they go to bed—the worst time they could be eating that stuff.

5) Help is only a click away. The Internet makes your food log more useful and easier to manipulate than ever before. Download your dietary information and various sites will analyze the nutritional profile.

listed will make a worthy substitute. Or if you hate one of our sample meals, replace it with one you find more palatable.

While everything is modular, nothing is arbitrary. Jim and I have made every food and meal choice for some specific reason. For example, grapefruit pops up frequently in our meal plans, and that's with good reason. New research from Scripps shows that subjects who ate several halves of grapefruit a day lost more weight than subjects who didn't—without even dieting!

The following sample meal plans represent what I typically eat. If you weigh less than 175 pounds, you'll want to reduce your intake. One way to do this is to cut out one of the three daily snacks. For example, if you don't feel hungry between breakfast and lunch, skip the late morning snack. Alternatively, you can reduce your intake by using smaller serving sizes for some meals. To cut back on protein, for example, eat two eggs instead of four at breakfast. You can also add less deli meat to sandwiches, or eat a smaller portion of protein (chicken, turkey, fish, steak) at dinner. To cut back on your carbohydrate intake, eat ½ a cup of cereal instead of 1 cup, ½ an English muffin, a small sweet potato instead of a large one, and ½ cup of rice or pasta instead of 1 cup.

Workout Eats

What's happening in the gym is important, but what you eat throughout the day can make the difference between success and failure. I'm inclined to agree with that perspective, based on my personal experience. That's why I drink my favorite protein shake, Isopure, as soon as I set down my last weight. They're quick, easy, and ready to drink.

It doesn't have to be a protein shake, but you should adopt the same habit of refueling your energy stores and feeding your muscles after exercising them. So on training days, consume one of these snacks as soon as possible after your workout.

Food	Calories	Protein (g)	Carbs (g)	Fat (g)
Power Bar Protein Plus	270	22	30	9
Clif Builder	270	20	30	8
16 oz. Jamba Juice Protein Berry Workout w/ soy protein	280	14	56	1
16 oz low-fat chocolate milk	316	16	52	4
8 oz plain nonfat yogurt + 1 cup blueberries	210	14	38	0

Sample Daily Meal Plans: Phase I
Monday

Breakfast
> 2 whole eggs
> 2 egg whites
> *Fry or scramble using non-fat cooking spray.*
>
> 1 whole-grain waffle, toasted
> 1 cup sliced strawberries
> 1 tablespoon fat-free sour cream
> 1 teaspoon brown sugar or plain table sugar
> *Mix sugar into sour cream. Add strawberries to waffle and top with sour cream mixture.*

Late-morning snack
> 1 cup plain low-fat yogurt
> ¼ cup granola
> *Mix granola into yogurt.*
>
> ½ large grapefruit

Lunch

4 ounces turkey deli meat

1 tablespoon light mayonnaise

2 slices whole-wheat bread

Lettuce and tomato slices (optional)

Spread mayo on bread and add turkey, along with lettuce and tomato if desired.

½ large grapefruit

Mid-afternoon snack

1 cup cottage cheese

½ cup sliced pineapple

6 whole-wheat crackers

Mix pineapple with cottage cheese and eat by scooping mixture up with crackers.

Dinner

8 ounces chicken breast

Bake, broil, or grill chicken with desired herbs or spices. at 350°F for 30 to 35 minutes.

1 large sweet potato

1 tablespoon fat-free sour cream

Butter substitute (optional)

Top sweet potato with sour cream and/or butter substitute.

1 cup broccoli

Steam or boil broccoli, or sauté in a tablespoon of olive oil, and sprinkle with 1 tablespoon Romano cheese as it cooks.

1 cup blueberries

2 tablespoons fat-free Reddi Wip

Top blueberries with Reddi Wip.

Late-night snack

1 cup skim milk

7 walnut halves

1 tablespoon peanut butter

Use peanut butter like a dip.

Totals: 2,246 calories, 243 grams of carbohydrates, 179 grams of protein, 65 grams of fat

* If you work out today, choose one snack from "Workout Eats," and consume within one hour of working out. Be sure to consider these nutritional values when planning your nutrition totals for the day.

Tuesday

Breakfast

1 cup skim milk

1 cup Kashi GoLean Cereal

Pour milk over cereal.

Late-morning snack

"Cobb" salad

2 cups mixed green salad

2 hard-boiled eggs, sliced

¼ cup dry oatmeal

¼ avocado, sliced

1 tablespoon low-fat ranch dressing

Top the greens with eggs, oatmeal, avocado, and dressing.

Lunch

4 ounces lean ground beef (95% lean)

1 whole-wheat hamburger bun

1 tablespoon catsup, mustard, or low-fat or fat-free mayo

Lettuce and sliced tomato (optional)

Mold ground beef into a patty. Cook in a pan or on a grill until done and place in bun. Add lettuce and tomato if desired.

1 cup cooked mixed vegetables (frozen or canned)

Mid-afternoon snack

Cheese quesadilla

10-inch whole-wheat tortilla

½ cup fat-free shredded cheddar cheese

Add cheese to one side of tortilla, fold in half, cook in frying pan over medium heat with 1 tablespoon olive oil on both sides until cheese is melted.

Dinner

6 ounces salmon (broiled or grilled)

1 cup cooked brown rice

1 cup canned, frozen, or fresh green beans (boiled or steamed)

½ cup jarred, canned, or fresh peach halves (the canned version should say "in its own juice"—avoid added sugar and syrup)

2 tablespoons fat-free Reddi Wip

Top peaches with Reddi Wip.

Late-night Snack

1 cup cottage cheese

2 tablespoon salsa

Top cottage cheese with salsa.

Totals: 2,106 calories, 226 grams of carbohydrates, 168 grams protein, 54 grams of fat

* If you work out today, choose one snack from "Workout Eats," and consume within one hour of working out. Be sure to consider these nutritional values when planning your nutrition totals for the day.

Wednesday

Breakfast

Cheese omelet
2 whole eggs
2 egg whites
¼ cup ricotta cheese (part skim)
¼ cup fat-free shredded mozzarella
Whisk eggs, pour in pan over medium heat with fat-free cooking spray, add cheeses, and fold eggs into omelet.

1 whole-wheat English muffin
1 teaspoon peanut butter
Spread peanut butter on English muffin.

Late-morning snack
1 cup boiled soybeans (edamame)
1 cup chicken noodle soup

Lunch
3 ounces tuna
1 tablespoon light mayonnaise
1 large wheat pita bread
Pickle relish and chopped celery (optional)
Mix tuna with mayo, add 1 tablespoon of pickle relish and diced celery if desired, spread into pita bread.

½ large grapefruit

Mid-afternoon snack
Wendy's Black Forest Ham and Swiss Frescata sandwich (no cheese)

Dinner
Turkey & vegetable pasta
4 ounces lean ground turkey
1 cup whole-wheat pasta
¼ cup jarred marinara sauce, heated (< 2 grams fat per serving)
1 cup sliced zucchini, steamed
Boil the pasta to desired softness, brown the turkey in pan, and then throw the turkey, sauce, and zucchini over the pasta.

2 squares (2 ounces) dark chocolate (60–70% cacao)
1 teaspoon peanut butter

Late-night snack
1 stick light mozzarella string cheese (1 ounce)
2 ounces beef jerky

Totals: 2,234 calories, 220 grams of carbohydrates, 178 grams of protein, 78 grams of fat

＊ If you work out today, choose one snack from "Workout Eats," and consume within one hour of working out. Be sure to consider these nutritional values when planning your nutrition totals for the day.

Thursday

Breakfast

Breakfast sandwich

2 whole eggs

1 slice low-fat American cheese

2 slices (2 ounces) low-fat deli ham

1 whole-wheat English muffin

Toast muffin; fry ham in pan and place on one half of muffin; fry eggs in pan, using non-stick cooking spray, and place on ham; top eggs with cheese and cover with other muffin half.

Late-morning snack

1 ounce (1/4 cup) shelled pumpkin seeds (pepitas)

1 cup container low-fat fruit yogurt

Lunch

6-inch Subway Turkey (double meat) on wheat with mustard and your choice of vegetables

Mid-afternoon snack

Cheese quesadilla

10-inch whole-wheat tortilla

1/2 cup fat-free shredded cheddar cheese

1 tablespoon olive oil (optional)

Add cheese to one side of tortilla, fold in half, cook in frying pan over medium heat with fat-free cooking spray or olive oil on both sides until cheese is melted.

Dinner

6 ounces top sirloin steak

1/2 cup black beans

1/2 cup brown rice

Broil or grill steak until it reaches desired doneness. Mix beans into rice.

1 cup sliced strawberries

1 tablespoon fat-free sour cream

1 teaspoon brown sugar or table sugar

Mix sour cream and sugar. Top strawberries with mixture.

Late-night snack

1 cup cottage cheese

2 tablespoons salsa

Top cottage cheese with salsa.

Totals: 2,053 calories, 227 grams of carbohydrates, 178 grams of protein, 50 grams of fat.

* If you work out today, choose one snack from "Workout Eats," and consume within one hour of working out. Be sure to consider these nutritional values when planning your nutrition totals for the day.

Friday

Breakfast

1 cup low-fat cottage cheese

1 cup fresh or canned mandarin oranges (the canned version should say "in its own juice"—avoid added sugar or syrup)

Mix oranges into cottage cheese.

2–3 large celery stalks

1 tablespoon peanut butter

Spoon peanut butter into the groove of the celery.

Late-morning snack

1 cup skim milk

1 cup Kashi GoLean Cereal

Pour milk over cereal.

Lunch

Turkey wrap

4 ounces turkey deli meat

1 slice low-fat American cheese

1 tablespoon light mayonnaise

10-inch whole-wheat tortilla

Warm tortilla if desired. Place turkey and cheese in middle of tortilla and spread with mayo. Roll up.

Late-afternoon snack

2 ounces fat-free cheese (Swiss, cheddar, Monterey jack, etc.)

9 whole-wheat crackers

Dinner

6 ounces tilapia (broiled or grilled)

½ cup black beans

1 whole-wheat dinner roll

1 cup blueberries

2 tablespoons fat-free Reddi Wip

Top blueberries with Reddi Wip

Late-night snack

1 stick light mozzarella string cheese (1 ounce)

1 cup skim milk

1 packet Swiss Miss fat-free cocoa mix

Warm milk in microwave or pan. Add cocoa mix and blend.

I like this combination. Then again, I like popcorn with M&Ms! In your case, feel free to eat the cheese and drink the hot chocolate separately.

Totals: 1,914 calories, 217 grams of carbohydrates, 172 grams of protein, 44 grams of fat.

✳ If you work out today, choose one snack from "Workout Eats," and consume within one hour of working out. Be sure to consider these nutritional values when planning your nutrition totals for the day.

Saturday

Breakfast

Veggie frittata

2 whole eggs

2 egg whites

$\frac{1}{4}$ cup low-fat cottage cheese

$\frac{1}{2}$ cup chopped broccoli

$\frac{1}{2}$ medium onion

In frying pan on medium heat, cook onions for about 5 minutes with fat-free cooking spray. Add broccoli and cook for about 5 minutes. In a bowl, beat eggs and cottage cheese, and add them to the pan. Lift and rotate the pan so that the eggs are evenly distributed. As eggs set around the edges, lift them to allow uncooked portions to flow underneath. Turn heat to low, cover the pan, and cook until top is set. Invert onto a plate.

1 packet Lower Sugar Quaker Instant Oatmeal (flavored: maple and brown sugar or apples and cinnamon)

Late-morning snack

1 cup plain low-fat yogurt

1 cup blueberries

Mix blueberries into yogurt.

Lunch

Ham sandwich

4 slices (4 ounces) low-fat deli ham

1 tablespoon light mayonnaise

2 slices whole-wheat bread

Lettuce and sliced tomato (optional)

Spread bread with mayo and add turkey. Top with lettuce and tomato if desired.

$\frac{1}{2}$ large grapefruit

Mid-afternoon snack

McDonald's Premium Grilled Chicken Classic (without mayo)

Dinner

Shrimp fried rice

4 ounces shrimp

1 large egg, beaten

1 cup brown rice, cooked

1 cup mixed frozen vegetables

1 tablespoon low-sodium soy sauce (optional)

In a pan over medium heat, cook shrimp in non-fat cooking spray. Add rice and vegetables; and egg and soy sauce, if desired. Cook for 5 to 10 minutes.

2 squares (2 ounces) dark chocolate (60–70% cacao)

1 teaspoon peanut butter

Late-night snack

Tzatziki

1 cup reduced-fat Greek yogurt (2%)

$\frac{1}{2}$ medium cucumber (peeled and diced)

Top cucumber wedges with yogurt.

Totals: 2,139 calories, 242 grams of carbohydrates, 167 grams of protein, 55 grams of fat.

* If you work out today, choose one snack from "Workout Eats," and consume within one hour of working out. Be sure to consider these nutritional values when planning your nutrition totals for the day.

Sunday

Breakfast

Ham & cheese omelet

2 whole eggs

2 egg whites

2 slice low-fat deli ham

¼ cup fat-free shredded cheddar cheese

Beat eggs and pour into heated pan with non-fat cooking spray. Sprinkle with cheese, add ham, and fold over eggs to make an omelet.

1 small low-fat bran muffin

Late-morning snack

1 cup plain low-fat yogurt

1 cup blueberries

Mix blueberries into yogurt.

Lunch

6-inch Subway Oven Roasted Chicken (double meat) on wheat, with your choice of any Subway vegetables as toppings

Mid-afternoon snack

Chicken salad

3 ounces canned chicken breast

1 tablespoon light mayonnaise

9 whole-wheat crackers

Mix mayo into chicken breast. Spread on crackers.

Dinner

Chicken & broccoli pasta

6 ounces chicken breast

1 cup whole-wheat pasta

¼ cup jarred marinara sauce (< 2 grams fat per serving)

1 cup chopped broccoli, steamed

Chop chicken and brown it in a pan using non-fat cooking spray or 1 tablespoon olive oil. After pasta is boiled, place on plate. Add chicken and broccoli and top with sauce.

2 cups mixed green salad

1 tablespoon low-fat ranch dressing

2 squares (2 ounces) dark chocolate (60–70% cacao)

1 teaspoon peanut butter

Late-night snack

1 cup cottage cheese

2 tablespoons salsa

Top cottage cheese with salsa.

Totals: 2,126 calories, 226 grams of carbohydrates, 197 grams of protein, 58 grams of fat.

✳ If you work out today, choose one snack from "Workout Eats," and consume within one hour of working out. Be sure to consider these nutritional values when planning your nutrition totals for the day.

QUICK & TASTY MEALS

Breakfast
Morning Smoothie

1 banana
1 tablespoon almond butter
1 tablespoon wheat germ
2½ scoops protein powder (such as Designer Protein)
½ cup orange juice
½ cup water and crushed ice

Add all ingredients to blender and blend until smooth. Add as much crushed ice as desired.

Makes 1 serving.

Total: 536 calories; 53 grams protein, 51 grams carbohydrates, 14.5 grams fat (29% protein, 37% carbohydrates, 24% fat)

Lunch & Dinner
1,000 calories
Oriental Beef and Vegetables

1 pound lean flank steak, fat trimmed
⅓ cup canned no-salt-added beef broth, undiluted
3 tablespoons low-sodium soy sauce
1 teaspoon sugar
1 teaspoon cornstarch
2 tablespoons peanut oil
⅓ pound fresh broccoli (washed, trimmed, head cut into florets, stalk in ⅓-inch slices)
2 cups sliced leeks
1 package pre-sliced fresh mushrooms
⅓ cup thinly sliced onion
8 cups torn fresh spinach
4 cups cooked long-grain rice (cooked without salt or fat)

Partially freeze steak. Slice diagonally across grain into ¼-inch strips. Set aside. Combine broth, soy sauce, sugar and cornstarch in a bowl; stir well. Set aside. Add oil to a wok or large nonstick skillet; place over medium heat until hot. Add steak and stir-fry 1 minute. Add reserved broth mixture; cover and simmer 2 minutes. Add broccoli, leeks, mushrooms, and onion; stir well. Place spinach on top of mixture; cover and cook 10 minutes or until spinach wilts and other vegetables are crisp-tender. Serve over cooked rice.

Makes 4 servings.

Add 2 cups egg drop soup; 1 sliced orange; 2 low-fat fig cookies; water or Crystal Light.

Total: 1,004 calories; 54 grams protein, 133 grams carbohydrates, 29 grams fat (21% protein, 53% carbohydrates, 26% fat)

Lunch & Dinner
500 calories

Turkey Burgers

Vegetable cooking spray
$\frac{1}{2}$ pound freshly ground raw turkey
$\frac{1}{2}$ cup chopped celery
$\frac{1}{4}$ cup chopped onion
1 can (8 ounces) no-salt-added tomato sauce
$\frac{3}{4}$ cup water
2 tablespoons toasted wheat germ
2 tablespoons tomato paste
2 teaspoon chili powder
$\frac{1}{8}$ teaspoon salt
$\frac{1}{8}$ teaspoon garlic powder
$\frac{1}{8}$ teaspoon ground cumin
6 ($1\frac{1}{2}$ ounces) whole-wheat buns
$\frac{1}{2}$ cup (2 ounces) shredded low-fat cheddar cheese
$\frac{1}{2}$ cup shredded lettuce

Coat a nonstick skillet with cooking spray; place over medium heat until hot. Add turkey, celery, and onion; cook until turkey is browned, stirring to crumble. Stir in tomato sauce, water, wheat germ, tomato paste, chili powder, salt, garlic powder, and ground cumin. Bring to a boil; cover and reduce heat and simmer for 10 minutes, stirring occasionally. Divide turkey mixture evenly between bottom halves of buns, top with shredded cheese, lettuce, and tops of buns.

Makes 6 servings.

Add 2 cups tossed salad; 2 tablespoons fat-free Italian salad dressing; 5 ounces boiled corn on the cob; $\frac{1}{2}$ cup grapes; water or Crystal Light.

Total: 505 calories; 26 grams protein, 82 grams carbohydrates, 9 grams fat (20% protein, 65% carbohydrates, 16% fat)

Snack

Yogurt Parfait

$\frac{1}{2}$ cup fat-free yogurt
$\frac{1}{2}$ cup fresh strawberries
1 tablespoon honey

137 calories; $4\frac{1}{2}$ grams protein; 30 grams carbohydrates; $\frac{1}{3}$ gram fat (13% protein; 86% carbohydrates; 1% fat)

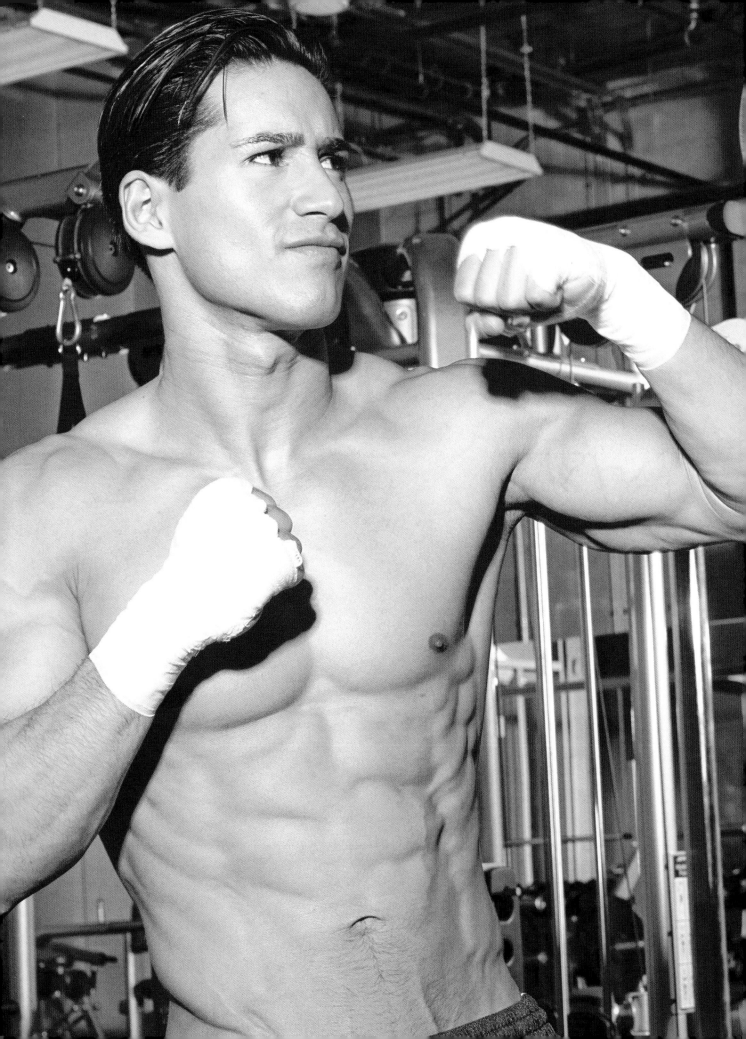

4 Staying Focused— It's All in Your Head

Many people hate going to the gym. They hem. They haw. They procrastinate. The very thought of lifting a weight fills them with dread.

They would hate me. I *love* working out. What's cool is that I feel like I can just set aside everything that has happened that day, good or bad, and escape inside the gym. That's my sanctuary, my decompression chamber, a place where I always feel happy and at home. That's why I always say that working out is the greatest stress reliever of all time. If you want to keep your head level and your mind focused, no pill, tranquilizer, or meditation technique comes close to blasting out a righteous workout, in my opinion.

Working out has really gotten me through the last five years. I've been blessed to work so much professionally, but it's also been stressful juggling so much. Training is so therapeutic for me because it clears my head and gives me the energy to keep up with it all. It's also a diversion and an escape from everything I've got going on. Mentally, physically, emotionally—it helps me with deal with whatever life sends my way.

For me, it's never been a question of being too busy to train. At least I don't think of it in that light. And, trust me, I'm as busy as anyone pretty much every single day of the year. I'm writing this at a desk in a hotel room in Las Vegas, where they just christened a brand-new studio at the Planet Hollywood Hotel for a show I work on, *Extra!* As soon as that wraps, I'm off to tape a special program for *Dancing with the Stars*.

Then I head off to do some last-minute voice-overs for a television movie I have coming up. After that, I fill in for the legendary host Larry King on his talk show. Then I board a plane and do a personal appearance, and then another one after that. Then I head to San Diego to host a charity event.

So, what did *you* do today?

My travel schedule is one reason I mix it up in the gym. I would go so far as to say that change is the watchword when it comes to my workouts. That's why sometimes I dance, and sometimes I box, although I always try to hit the weights, do body-weight exercises, or do several a few times a week. Those are my staples. It would be easy to blow off my workouts, but I don't do *easy*. In fact, the workouts, in large measure, are what allow me to accomplish everything I just outlined. As I've said many times before, the mental approach to exercise is huge. Think about it: Why do you have great workouts sometimes—and know you're about to have a great one as soon as you exit your car to enter the gym? And how do you think your fitness level and physical shape would be affected if you had more of those types of workouts, more of the time?

Is there a special secret to experiencing these amazing workouts? Some magic motivational pill enabling you to become mentally zoned, so you naturally exert consistent, determined, high-energy workout efforts? That's what we're going to explore in this chapter: the mental game.

Here's the thing about the functional and old-school camps sniping back and forth, which we discussed in Chapter 1: Heck, at least they're all working out! The key to not only shaping up, but also to staying in shape once you're there, is sticking with the program even as other aspects of your life attempt to crowd it out. And, trust me, this assault is continuous. Any number of scenarios can result in people falling off the workout wagon, and I'm going to outline 10 that I've noticed over the years:

1) **Diving in without adequate information, understanding, and mental preparation.** Then finding out it's either more than you realized or not what you expected.

2) **Procrastination.** Always finding a reason to put off working out to another day.

3) **Lack of commitment.** Everyone has days when they don't feel like working out, including me. But these people lack consistency of passion, effort, or even intent.

   Often I see this happening after my friends get married. I tell those guys, "Dude, you need to give your wife a visual! If you want a visual, you've got to give a visual!" I tease 'em a little about it.

4) **Relying too much on external motivation and the encouragement of others.** Lacking it, this person instinctively falls back on the status quo: the couch.

5) **Lack of attention.** If recognition and praise aren't forthcoming, this person loses interest and motivation. He or she thinks, *If I have no one to perform for or impress, so what's the point?*

6) **Lack of long-term commitment.** This person thinks, *I wanted it when I wanted it, but I thought it would happen sooner!* When success doesn't happen, like, yesterday, they raise the white flag.

7) **Low self-esteem and self-image.** This person sabotages initial success by thinking, I feel like I'm not supposed to amount to anything. I'm not supposed to be somebody.

8) **Need for a specific event or external motivation.** These people will kill themselves to look good for a wedding, high school reunion, speaking engagement, or photo shoot. But take away the upcoming event, and they lose their motivation and discipline.

9) **Allowing less-than-ideal conditions to sour their attitude.** When this person can't find a quick parking space, can't handle the crowd in the health club, can't stand waiting for equipment, can't stand hearing people talking around them, it's not just a minor imperfection. It's a reason to throw in the towel.

10) **Unrealistic expectations.** This person thinks fitness success will happen overnight, instead of understanding that it's a long-range process, and that mastering the process takes time.

One way to stay on the workout wagon is to learn more about training and dieting, and purchasing this book was a great start. Knowledge makes it easier to work out when you're traveling or staring down crazy deadlines. You'll learn how to make your workouts shorter but more intense, producing the same results in less time. In the meantime, feel free to use one of the special 10-minute workouts, scattered throughout this book, when you lack enough time to give one of the regular workouts your complete and undivided attention. But make those days the exception, not the rule.

The key thing is still doing *something* physical, even when your schedule is slammed six ways till Sunday. To use a traffic metaphor, it's okay to be stuck at a red light—just don't park your car and wander away, or you might get lost. Even if you're having a really bad, really crazy week, stay connected to your workouts rather than give up on them. The end-of-year holidays offer a classic example. During those two or three weeks around Christmas, you're probably going to miss some workouts while you're visiting family or whatever. It happens to all of us. But even if you can squeeze in one or two workouts, you're staying connected. You're not losing focus completely. It's no problem to tread water during tough stretches. Just don't go under.

People stay connected to their fitness in different ways. I hear a lot about how a training partner makes it easier to stick with the program, and I have no doubt that's true. A study published in *The Journal of Sports Medicine and Physical Fitness* found that when married couples exercise together, they have higher attendance and lower dropout rates than singles shaping up solo. That's cool—a nice added benefit to having someone special in your life; couples that train together remain together. Anytime you can share the same interests with your partner, it strengthens your relationship.

Other people say one of the main reasons they employ the services of a personal trainer is not so much the expertise they receive, but the encouragement it gives them to show up (especially when it's either show up, or pay a hefty cancellation fee!). And, hey, take it from the host of Animal Planet's *Pet Star*—your best workout partner might even train on four legs. In a random phone survey, whose subjects were chosen at random University of Victoria researchers found that dog owners exercise twice as much as those lacking canine companionship. If you've ever owned a dog (I don't have one now, but I'm planning to get one soon) you know how pushy and demanding they can be when it comes time to head out for their daily exercise. We should all be so disciplined and determined!

I've trained with a partner, and I also have a personal trainer, the aforementioned Jimmy Peña, the Texas Tornado, who knows exercise backwards, forwards, and sideways. That being said, everyone needs to be able to train alone if they're going to succeed in the long term. Sometimes your training partner or personal trainer won't be available, and you can't miss a workout every time that happens.

The bigger issue, however, is the need for self-motivation rather than external motivation. What's an external motivator? Shaping up so you look good in your wedding dress. A bet with a friend to see who can lose the most weight. A personal trainer jaw-jacking you to show up for your workout. Here are a few external reasons people use to begin working out that typically spell doom:

1) **Feeling guilty.** Thinking, I should be doing something about being out of shape.
2) **Being heavily influenced by societal trends and peer pressures.**

Feeling an intense need to conform, to measure up to standards, to be like everyone else.

3) **Doing it to please, impress, or satisfy someone else.** Thinking, *Oh, my wife/husband wants me to get into shape,* or *Oh, the people in my office were making comments about me having gained weight,* or, *Oh, the people at my beach club, social club, organization look better than I do, so it's time for me to take action.*

Bottom line: You need to *want* to do it. You have to find the reason (or reasons) that you want to improve your body and your life. Instead of wondering with dread when you can spare 30 minutes for a workout, you need to reach the point where you think, *I could go to the movies or restaurant right now . . . only I would rather work out. That sounds like more fun to me right now.* When that becomes your thought process—look out, world! The great body, the six-pack abs, the spring in your step—all of that good stuff will surely follow. And there's nothing I love more than seeing that happen in real life.

I've turned a lot of people onto the boxing gym, and I've prompted others who aren't necessarily into punching things to hit the regular gym for the first time in their life. Whatever they want to try, I encourage them to go for it. When they start losing weight, they feel better, as do I, watching the whole process unfold before my eyes. It's all about motivating each other, pushing each other, and it's neat to behold. Most of them have kept it up, too. That in turn inspires me.

Even girls I've gone out with in the past who maybe weren't into fitness got into it from my encouragement. All my ex-girlfriends look hotter than they did when I was going out with them because I got them into working out. We broke up—and they kept training. You guys owe me!

So if you need to train with a partner, find one. If you like to train solo, go it alone. The best approach to choose is the one that is most likely to propel you into the gym or onto a treadmill.

That's the bigger picture: Staying the course for the duration of this workout program and beyond, until working out and eating right are so firmly ingrained in your psyche that you never think about not working out. Failure? Not an option. That is what people mean when they talk about fitness becoming part of your lifestyle. It certainly has become an important part of mine. What I can't impress upon you enough is the cumulative power of working out and eating right. Waking up one day and deciding that you need to go the gym because you're not happy with yourself means nothing. That's like deciding to learn

Spanish and taking one class. But make that small investment every day, and you'll become a different person. One year from now, or two years from now, you'll think, *I can't imagine not having done this! It's opened up so many more possibilities for me in life.*

But it's not the entire picture. The devil is in the details, as they say, and you also have to wring every benefit out of each individual workout. I love the Chinese expression that states: "A journey of a thousand miles begins with a single step." Your journey, the one to becoming physically fit, begins with a single rep with a dumbbell and your next step on the treadmill. Make it an amazing rep and an amazing step! Without going all Zen on you, I believe it's important—no, essential—to cultivate the mindset that every single workout is critically important to achieving overall success. Will some workouts of necessity wind up being better than others? Yes, of course they will. There are intangibles that we can't always control, and they can help or hinder us. It could be something as simple and random as an amazing song coming over the gym's loudspeakers just when you need to dig deep for that last rep. But you don't want hit the gym door thinking you'll simply go through the motions and then mail it in. Those don't count in my workout book.

University of Iowa researchers recently found that people who stick with their weight-loss plan tend to be the ones who concentrate on specific *actions* rather than on the desired results. What does that mean for you? Let's say your goal is shedding 15 pounds of fat by the time your high school reunion rolls around. Don't obsess over the magic number—15 pounds, 15 pounds, 15 pounds—or an upcoming event like a high school reunion or your wedding. Instead, you're much better off making a list of 10 concrete actions that will contribute to achieving that end result. For example, every day, when 11 a.m. rolls around and the pre-lunch munchies hit, grab a handful of almonds from your desk and drink a cup of green tea instead of feeding the vending machine. That one small change will make a huge difference over time, especially if it's only one of 10 similarly small yet important changes.

HEY, MARIO!

I'm working out but my loved ones aren't supporting me like I expected them to. In fact, some of them are openly hostile. What should I do?

You shaping up will threaten certain people in your life, even those with whom you're closest. You're changing and they're not. Deep down, they may be wondering how this will affect your relationship over time. It's a valid concern, even if they're not aware of it and are just projecting. Encourage them to join you in this effort, and don't let them discourage you from yours. In the end it's their problem, not yours.

That's what I do. I always put together game plans and blueprints not only for what I want to achieve but also for how I intend to accomplish it. I'm like a cartographer: I love mapping things out—Plan A, Plan B, and so on down the line. I'll formulate as many plans as I need to finish the job. The planning process isn't a chore for me. I love to write everything down. I love to have a game plan. I love to be very organized. I love to have everything scheduled. I'd feel right at home in the military, where everything is regimented.

You need to be psyching yourself up before you ever enter the gym—which for me is usually first thing in the morning. (Unless I'm boxing that day. The last thing anyone wants to do is wake up and get punched in the nose even before they've had their morning coffee.) Those of you who learn how to take yourselves mentally and emotionally to the place you really want to be *before you ever touch the weights* are the ones who will be the most successful. That's one positive lesson you can learn from champion bodybuilders. By the time those guys pick up their first weight, they've already had an amazing workout in their mind. Success will follow because they've practiced it mentally.

While you're changing into your gym clothes, take time to run through a series of images in your mind. Your images will be different from mine or anyone else's, but they should have something to do with relaxing physically, and then focusing all of your mental energy on the task ahead, the same way I need to focus before I step on stage. Ideally, the image should remind you of your long-term goal, and confirm that this upcoming workout is another pinpoint on the road map leading to your destination. Even if you're having a bad day, mired in difficulty, muttering negative thoughts to yourself over and over, think about how much better you will feel about yourself if you complete *this one workout* out instead of blowing it off. Working out is more powerful than any drug at combating life's challenges. You're fighting back, not surrendering.

Once you enter the gym doors, maintaining your focus isn't easy, trust me. As a celebrity, I'm prone to being recognized there, and people often seek me out. Most of the time, I love interacting with my fans. I'm a natural talker anyway, which you probably already know if you've seen me hosting beauty pageants on TV. But when I'm there to work out, I like to just go in and say to myself "Okay, are you ready now?" Asking myself that question is like a mental cueing mechanism, telling me that it's "go" time. That allows me to focus and lock in that feeling. I might not say another word for the next hour.

Anyone who knows what they're doing in the gym is subject to attention, including questions. It's what people do. They see somebody who looks like they know what they're doing, so they want to pick their brain. If you're the person being approached, you don't want to be anti-social, of course, but you need to strike a balance between answering the question and still proceeding to your next set. One way to maintain your momentum in the face of interruptions is to keep moving. If you need to, wear headphones and keep your eyes focused on the task at hand. If you're standing around, looking at other people, casting your gaze in different directions, you invite interaction. It's tricky, because I love people and hate to send off the message that I'm unapproachable or unfriendly. Because I'm not—anything but. So, when I first enter the gym, I'll spend a short amount of time smiling and shaking hands. But once my workout begins, I stay focused. I'm there to accomplish something! I'm in my training zone.

This doesn't come naturally to me. I have a very short attention span, probably shorter than yours, and I'll be the first to admit that. Like me, you need to learn what your own attention span is inside the gym. Wear a sports watch to your next workout and notice when your attention starts to lag. Many people working out can pay attention for 10, 15, maybe 20 minutes. They're really into it. But at some point, they lose their focus.

The rapid-fire nature of the workouts in this book reflect the rhythms of my own attention span, which is admittedly short—my mind wants to stray but my workouts are structured so that it can't. There's not a lot of down time, not a lot of pausing, very little sitting around. The pace goes boom, boom, boom. That's why I could never train like a power lifter, resting 3 to 5 minutes between sets. My mind would check out. Even during my brief rest periods in between sets, I keep moving.

In the case of your gym workout, when you do find yourself with brief breaks between sets or supersets, try taking a moment to close your eyes, breathe deeply, and remember a moment in time that felt really good, like sitting on a favorite stretch of beach. It will vary , but conjure an image that really allows you to relax. Then pick up your task again—the next set—with a fresh burst of energy and renewed attention. Allow yourself to focus intensely only when you're doing that set, and then let your mind wander. In fact, encourage your mind to drift a bit. That way you'll be fresh and ready for your next set.

Another thing that helps me stay focused during my workouts is really mastering each set and each repetition. I'm a real stickler for correct form, and if you're paying attention to form, you can't really pay attention to anything else. Remember, weights can lead to injury if you're not careful. You can pull a hamstring or damage your delicate shoulder joint if you lose focus on what you're doing. You're pushing iron around. Don't think you're invincible just because you're a young 'un, either. You're most likely to rupture your chest muscles in your 20s and 30s. Chalk it up to ego and machismo. Tears to the pectoralis major—your largest chest muscle—typically occur in men trying to bench-press more weight than they can handle, report Boston University researchers.

Where your head is focused during the set itself is again a matter of personal preference. Some people succeed by focusing, laser-like, on every muscle fiber firing during their rep. Others extend their set by placing some space between their mind and their body. After all, when lactic acid builds up in your muscle and "the burn" sets in like a five-alarm fire, your body likely will be telling your brain one thing: "What, are you crazy? Put down that weight!" I've talked to successful athletes who've taken both approaches. Some just tell themselves that they're going to focus on the last part of the rep and push themselves through it. Others describe it more as just letting go of themselves, almost like an out-of-body experience. "My body just took over from my brain," is the sort of thing they'll say.

There's no one-size-fits-all answer to this question, so I suggest figuring out what works best for you through trial and error. For your next few workouts, focus your attention intensely on the weights during your set. Then do a few workouts where you take the opposite approach. When you reach the make-or-break part of your set, let go with your mind and allow your body to take over. Imagine you're outside your body, watching it move the weight. Try each one of those approaches for several days, and soon you'll have your answer. Once you know which approach works for you, you can sharpen and ultimately perfect it.

All this stuff about being in "the zone" and achieving "peak performance" isn't magic. The information can be learned, the techniques practiced. If you do the mental work beforehand, you can get the most out of your body in the gym. Start with this mental warm-up, which I developed with Peter C. Siegel, RH.

HEY, MARIO!

I'm 30 now and I feel like I missed the boat on the whole getting in shape thing. What can I do?

I'm glad you asked this, because I'm 35—and in the best shape of my life! Here's what your age is: numbers on a birth certificate. Who cares? Sixty is the new 40, so you haven't even hit your prime yet. I don't even know if you're a man or woman, but it doesn't matter, because at that age, you still have the energy stores, metabolism, and hormonal environment needed to build an amazing body. The only thing you don't have is a bunch of time to waste. **So what are you waiting for?**

7 STEPS TO YOUR BEST WORKOUT EVER

1) Before you enter the gym, gently close your eyes, and draw in a long, deep breath through your nostrils. Then, slowly exhale through your mouth. Next, recall the very last workout where you knew and thoroughly felt you'd have a great workout—even before you started.

2) Once this memory becomes specific and clear, mentally step into the picture, and into your body. And then, let yourself think, feel, and breathe exactly the way you did before. Go ahead and *really* think about what you thought, feel what you felt, and breathe exactly the way you breathed. While you're doing that, choose one word (e.g., force, power, drive) that you feel represents you as the embodiment of this feeling. Mentally, silently exclaim it to yourself three consecutive times.

3) I want you to imaginatively experience yourself as the full embodiment of this feeling performing one full set of an exercise you'll be doing during your workout. You're not just "visualizing" here. You're purposefully engaging the exercise, and using the weight (or the movement) to directly work the muscle you're training through the full range of motion. Mentally exclaim your key word, then imaginatively engage your set, feeling yourself mentally locked in, determined, and totally working the body part you're training throughout each rep of the entire set.

4) Now, shift your awareness so that you're envisioning checking your body out in one of the gym mirrors. Clearly experience your body specifically reflecting the shape, detail, and proportion that your entire workout is geared to produce. Mentally experience yourself possessing and reflecting your desired end result . . . as if this specific physical shape, detail, and proportion is your reality, right *now*! As you're clearly envisioning yourself reflecting this peak, vital, physical shape, say to yourself (and *mean* it), "*This* is what my efforts today naturally compel me to bring forth; creating *this* physical shape fiercely energizes my determination—and commitment to prevail—right *now*!"

5) Slowly let your eyelids open, inhale deeply, grab your gym bag, and go!

6) After performing several times, this entire 1 through 5 process should take 3 to 4 minutes, hardly a high price to pay for moving yourself toward peak motivated effort, workout after workout. Each time you use this strategy as outlined, it will become steadily easier for you to perform, and your results will be ever more profound.

7) Be sure you properly warm up before engaging any workout; make this a rule of thumb. And I also encourage you to mentally exclaim your chosen key word before you perform each individual set of your workout. This will serve to reinforce a connection between purpose, mission, personal triumph, and your workout efforts.

Phase 2
Weeks
3 and 4

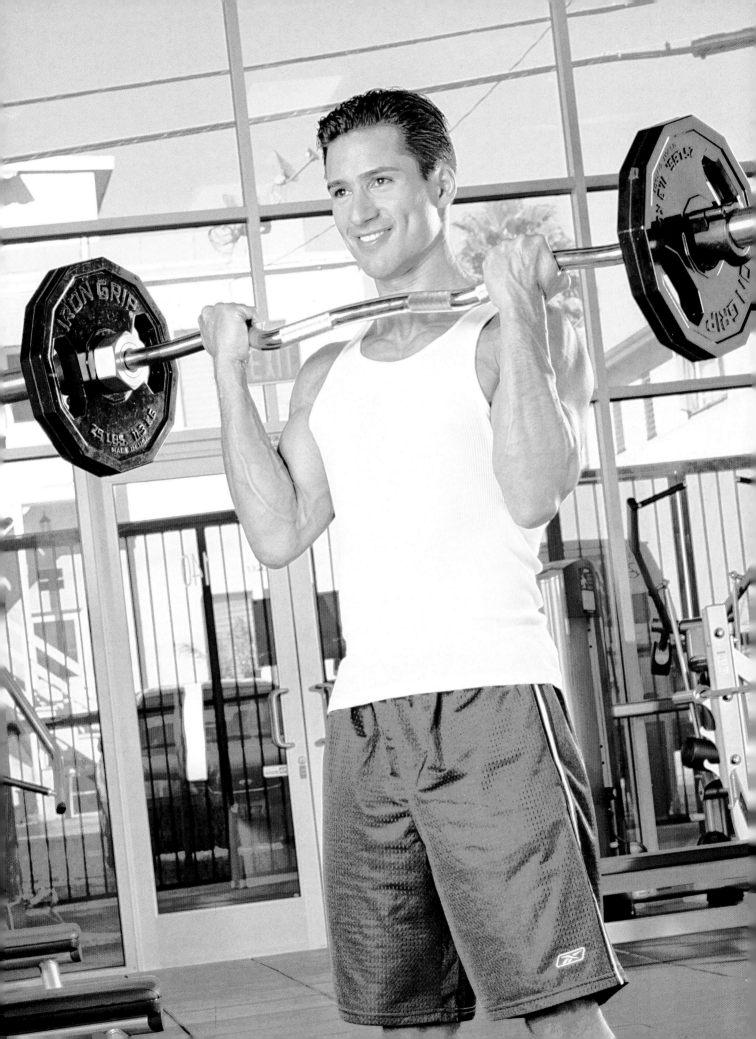

5 Fueling the Fire!

Now that you've finished two weeks of training (or four, if you were a beginner), congratulations are in order. I'd tell you to enjoy an amazing dinner out and a cocktail—that's what I do to celebrate a major achievement—but we're not there yet. After you've patted yourself on the back, don't rest on your laurels. It's time to get right back to work! Welcome to Phase II of my program designed to take you to the next level.

The gains you've made should already be starting to show, but don't be disappointed if the signs are only playing peek-a-boo with you at this early juncture. After all, there's still a ways to go and much more progress to be made. Even though you won't have six-pack abs after only two weeks, all sorts of great things are already happening beneath the surface of your skin. For starters, the pace dictated by those supersets and interval cardio has already begun setting layers of fat ablaze. What's more, you should already be experiencing noticeable improvements in energy and stamina, both in the gym and in your everyday life.

One thing you will never be when following my workouts is bored, and Phase II is Exhibit A in why that's true. You're still going to be performing exercises back to back with no rest in between; this time, however, we're going to add a third set to each grouping, making everything a little harder. Don't shy away from this, though. That's how the body improves. You subject yourself to workouts that are a little harder than the ones before it, and the body says, "Whoa, what's going on here? I need to adapt or I'm going to get buried!" I love it when my trainer pushes me through a particularly hard workout. I'm not sure I could reach that level on my own. I can tell when I've trained my butt off because I sleep so well that night. We trained so hard the other night that I felt like I slipped into a coma when I went to bed. Do the same workouts over and over again, and the body kicks back and puts its feet up on a chair. "Why sweat it?" the body says. After all, it's learned to handle those demands with the muscle power and the cardiovascular ability it already possesses. The good news is that the human body adapts very quickly to new training challenges. We were built for it.

The added challenge to your body goes beyond the presence of a third exercise of each trio or grouping. It's the *kind* of moves that I'm adding to the traditional strength training exercises. I start including some calisthenics that are great for general conditioning. Jumping jacks and skipping rope each take a bow before kicking your butt in Phase II. Some of you might not have done these exercises since gym class in grade school. But take it from a guy

6 TRAINING MISTAKES TO AVOID AT ALL COSTS

1) Overtraining. When we think of rest and recovery, we usually think of individual body-part training: *Let's see, I trained biceps on Tuesday, so I can hit them again on Friday.* But you also need to account for the central nervous and endocrine system, your energy stores, and so on. While you can give each body part enough rest, your body as as whole often gets too little. Give the whole system a rest, and stay out of the gym for a day or two sometimes.

2) Too many sets can equal failure. Sometimes it's good to keep going until you can't squeeze out another rep. But people go too far, which eventually leads back to Item 1: overtraining. Keep going after receiving a helping hand on one or two forced reps, and your partner ends up doing the work. It's just a waste of time, you know?

3) Locking out your elbows after pressing dumbbells or a barbell. When you lock out, you rest in the middle of a repetition and risk injury. Stop just short of locking out. We want your body to be saved by the dumbbells, not destroyed by them.

4) Relaxing on the negative. Beginners especially tend to focus on raising the weight, but lowering it is the most productive half of the rep. "Dropping" the weight back to the starting position also jeopardizes ligaments and tendons.

5) Thinking that only free weights are for going heavy. Many machines allow for going heavy and stimulating muscle fibers in a way that will make them grow—just as with free weights.

6) Endless repetition. Too many people find one routine that they like and stick with it indefinitely. Only the body grows accustomed to what it's being asked to do every single session and stops adapting. The result: stagnation. Your muscles should constantly be shocked with new movements.

who attended a real high school and a TV high school: Your gym teacher knew what he was doing, because they still work great.

I also appreciate their versatility. When you're traveling, or you can't make it to the gym for whatever reason, calisthenics moves can easily be arranged to form a complete workout. (And leave those M&Ms in the minibar while you're at it!)

I've stayed in dingy hotel rooms in the most out-of-the-way towns in America, and I've had to get really creative to bust a workout in those places. Sometimes it's too cold even to run, so I'll bring a jump rope, or some bands, or use the bed or chairs for a workout. I do pushups, situps, crunches, dips, stuff like that. Sometimes I'll go in the bathroom, let the hot water run until it gets real steamy, and shadow box for ten minutes for a quick cardio blast.

The weight workouts almost become like interval circuits, increasing the energy expenditure of each workout. Translation: You'll be burning even more calories than you were in Phase I. And you'll burn those calories with extreme efficiency, without wasting any time in the gym beyond what you need to shape up. As a general rule, that's how I like to amp up my workout intensity—by making sessions denser, rather than than by dragging them out. The research shows this approach really works: Exercise scientists at Smith College in Massachusetts found that raising your intensity probably does more for losing weight than how often you exercise, or for how long.

You'll also find more plyometrics moves (any exercise in which muscles are repeatedly and rapidly stretched and then contracted, like pushups, with a clap at the top of each rep) included in Phase II. Conventional bodybuilding exercises such as the bench press and squat) build muscle first and foremost, and plyometrics moves do that as well. In fact, the fast-twitch fibers that plyos use produce a lot of force in a short period of time, providing the greatest upside for making your muscles both bigger and more toned. They're genetically programmed for growth, which explains why sprinters, for example, showcase

HEY, MARIO!

If I lose my focus on a set in your workout, can I make it up by doing two more?

Avoid developing the mindset that instead of doing one set with the proper mental focus, you can make up for it by doing two or even three sloppier sets. You can't make up for lack of intensity with more volume. Intensity is what stimulates growth, so train accordingly. It saves time, too. Why do three sets when you can achieve the same or better results with one good one?

such amazingly well developed legs. And they offer a bonus: explosiveness. When you take to the basketball court for Workout D during this phase, you may have to alert air traffic control—your jumps will be that improved. The net result is that you'll be swishing shots with more athleticism and greater overall fitness.

As you learned in Phase I, cardio comes after the weight training, where it produces the best results. First, you don't want cardio to fatigue your muscles so much that by the time you pick up the weights, lifting effectively becomes a struggle. Unless cardio becomes your main focus for whatever reason, do that part *after* your rack the dumbbells. Strength training has less of a negative impact on cardio than cardio has on strength training. After all, with cardio, the goal is to elevate your heart rate, not win an Olympic gold medal in sprinting.

The benefits of my weights-first/cardio-second approach also extend to fat burning. As it turns out, weight training signals your body to release hormones whose job it is to signal the body to torch lard. I know this because Japanese scientists found that those who hit the weights and then work the stationary bike burn twice as much fat as those who only pedal.

I'm switching you from the stationary bike to the rower, however. Every cardio apparatus is capable of elevating your heart rate, but each machine works muscles in different ways. Let's take advantage of that variety. If you've been working the stationary cycle for months on end, and then hop on the treadmill one day—your body will shocked. Because the treadmill is unfamiliar, using it will seem much, much harder to your body. Cardio works best when it forces the body to adapt to new demands.

Aside from the mirror, what's the most accurate gauge of changes in your body on my program? You're right if you're focusing on muscle and fat— the ratio between the two is your "body composition." Unfortunately, neither your weight nor your body mass index (BMI) will reveal if you're more blubber than brawn. What's more, Japanese

HEY, MARIO!

A lot of your workout guidance (intervals, supersets, etc.) call for compressing more work into less time. Don't we lose some calorie burning by not working out as long?

Actually, no. Researchers have looked into this question, and as it turns out, you can completely trade duration for intensity. What's important is how many calories you burn—not the means by which you burn them. Personally, I like the efficiency of intervals.

researchers claim that bathroom scales claiming to measure body fat don't always account for the water content in your cells, yielding inflated percentages as a result.

If you want to be exact, try *hydrostatic weighing*, which is like a carnival dunk tank: You sit on a special scale that's then submerged in a tank of water. (They're typically offered at high-end health clubs, dieting organizations, and university metabolism labs. Your average gym or doctor's office likely won't have one.) Because of the difference in density between muscle and fat, the fat percentage is gleaned by applying a formula to the number on the scale. Aim for less than 18 percent if you're a guy and less than 25 percent if you're a woman.

PHASE II PRIMARY GOALS:
- ## More muscle
- ## Less fat
- ## Increased energy

Phase II

Beginner							
	Monday	Tuesday	Wednesday	Thursday	Friday	Saturday	Sunday
WEEK 1:	Workout A	Rest	Workout B	Rest	Workout A	Workout C	Rest
WEEK 2:	Workout B	Rest	Workout A	Rest	Workout B	Workout D	Rest
WEEK 3:	Workout A	Rest	Workout B	Rest	Workout A	Workout C	Rest
WEEK 4:	Workout B	Rest	Workout A	Rest	Workout B	Workout D	Rest
Intermediate and Advanced							
	Monday	Tuesday	Wednesday	Thursday	Friday	Saturday	Sunday
WEEK 1:	Workout A	Rest	Workout B	Workout C	Workout A	Workout D	Rest
WEEK 2:	Workout B	Rest	Workout A	Workout C	Workout B	Workout D	Rest

Phase II:
Workout A Weights and Cardio

Sequence	Week	Exercise	Sets[1]	Reps[2]	Rest[3]
A1	1	Dumbbell Squat	3	10–12	↓
	2	Dumbbell Squat	3	10–12	↓
	3	Dumbbell Squat	3	10–12	↓
	4	Dumbbell Squat	3	10–12	↓
A2	1	Swiss Ball Dumbbell Chest Press	3	10–12	↓
	2	Swiss Ball Dumbbell Chest Press	3	10–12	↓
	3	Swiss Ball Dumbbell Chest Press	3	10–12	↓
	4	Swiss Ball Dumbbell Chest Press	3	10–12	↓
A3	1	Jumping Jacks	3	25–50	60
	2	Jumping Jacks	3	25–50	60
	3	Jumping Jacks	3	25–50	60
	4	Jumping Jacks	3	25–50	60
B1	1	Dumbbell Romanian Deadlift	3	10–12	↓
	2	Dumbbell Romanian Deadlift	3	10–12	↓
	3	Dumbbell Romanian Deadlift	3	10–12	↓
	4	Dumbbell Romanian Deadlift	3	10–12	↓
B2	1	Barbell Row	3	10–12	↓
	2	Barbell Row	3	10–12	↓
	3	Barbell Row	3	10–12	↓
	4	Barbell Row	3	10–12	↓
B3	1	Squat Thrust	3	10–20	60
	2	Squat Thrust	3	10–20	60
	3	Squat Thrust	3	10–20	60
	4	Squat Thrust	3	10–20	60
C1	1	Dumbbell Lateral Raise	3	10–12	↓
	2	Dumbbell Lateral Raise	3	10–12	↓
	3	Dumbbell Lateral Raise	3	10–12	↓
	4	Dumbbell Lateral Raise	3	10–12	↓
C2	1	Lying Dumbbell Triceps Extension	3	10–12	↓
	2	Lying Dumbbell Triceps Extension	3	10–12	↓
	3	Lying Dumbbell Triceps Extension	3	10–12	↓
	4	Lying Dumbbell Triceps Extension	3	10–12	↓
C3	1	Mini-Trampoline Jogging	3	Up to 45 seconds	60
	2	Mini-Trampoline Jogging	3	Up to 45 seconds	60
	3	Mini-Trampoline Jogging	3	Up to 45 seconds	60
	4	Mini-Trampoline Jogging	3	Up to 45 seconds	60
D1	1	Cable Reverse Wood Chop	3	10–12/side	60
	2	Cable Reverse Wood Chop	3	10–12/side	60
	3	Cable Reverse Wood Chop	3	10–12/side	60
	4	Cable Reverse Wood Chop	3	10–12/side	60
E1		Rowing intervals: Row for 3 minutes at a easy pace, then perform 6–8 repetitions of 30–60 seconds each, followed by 90–120 seconds of rest.			

[1] Do modified supersets with each pair of exercises listed with the same number (for example, A1 and A2); that is, do the prescribed number of sets for each of the two exercises in alternating fashion before moving on to the next pairing. (For example, if the program calls for three sets, do one set of split squats followed by one set of push-ups, and then repeat twice). Rest in between each set as prescribed.

[2] The last rep you can finish with complete control and perfect form should fall within this range, so select your weight accordingly. Once you have completed all your repetitions with your current weight for two consecutive workouts, increase your poundage slightly. Five pounds for each new step is a good rule of thumb.

[3] Between supersets, measured in seconds.

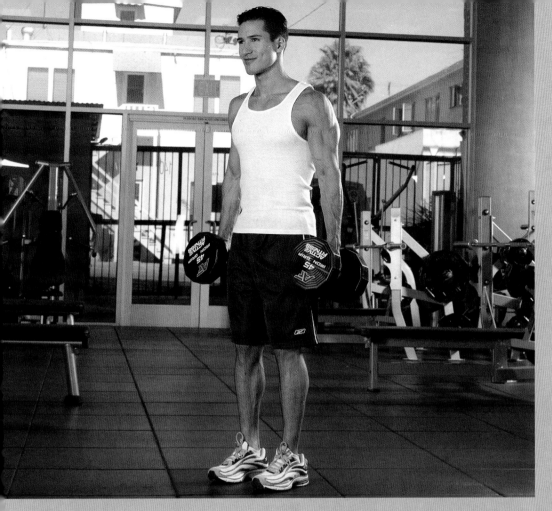

DUMBBELL SQUAT

Great for:
football, skiing

Get ready!

Stand with your feet shoulder-width apart holding a pair of dumbbells at your sides, palms facing each other.

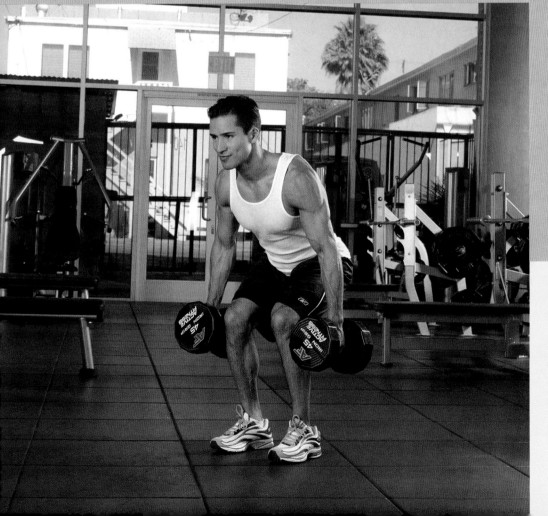

Go!

Imagine sitting down in a chair as you let your hips move back, lowering yourself until your thighs are parallel with the floor. Pause. Push yourself back up into a standing position.

Watch out for:

Back problems. Avoid them by keeping your back naturally arched throughout each repetition. Also watch for improper breathing. Inhale before you start a rep, and exhale when you complete it.

SWISS BALL DUMBBELL CHEST PRESS

Great for: boxing, baseball

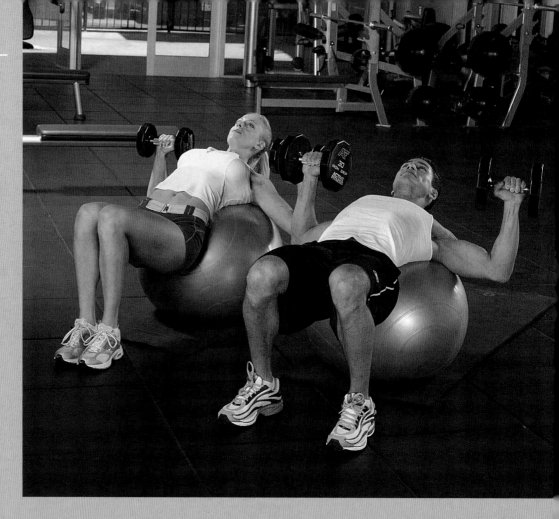

Get ready!

Lie face-up on a Swiss ball holding a pair of dumbbells out at your shoulders, palms facing forward.

Go!

Press the weights overhead in an arc until your arms are fully extended, at which point the dumbbells should nearly touch, yet still remain inches apart. Return to the starting position.

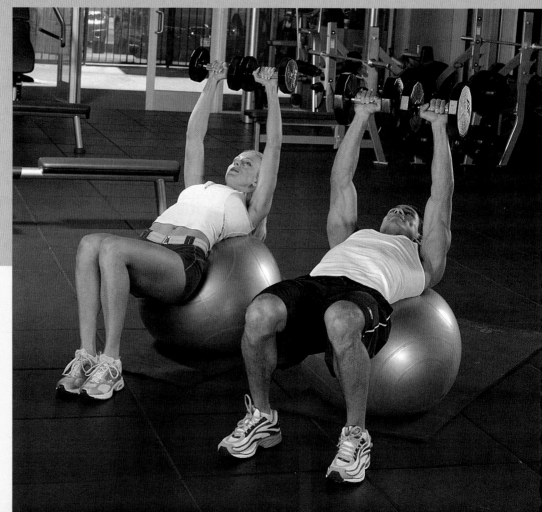

Watch out for:

To protect your shoulders, keep your shoulder blades pulled back and down as you raise and lower the weight.

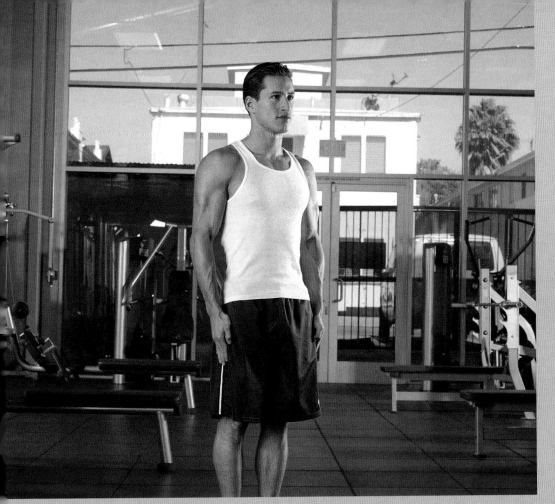

JUMPING JACK

Great for:
soccer, rugby

Get ready!

Stand straight with your hands at your sides and your feet nearly together.

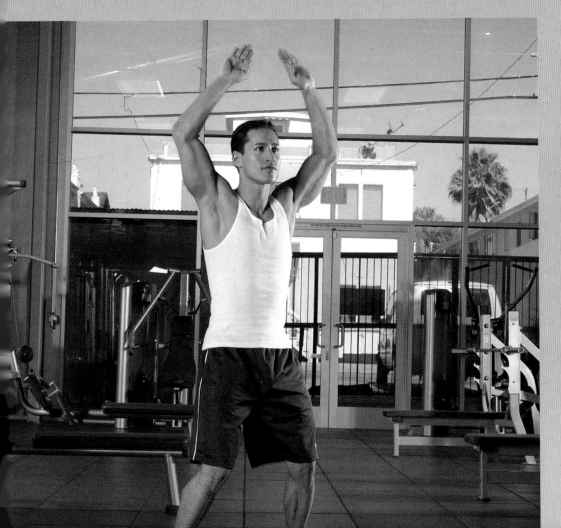

Go!

Jump and scissor-kick your legs out to the side, simultaneously bringing your hands together above you in an arc for a clap. Return to the starting position and repeat. The movement should be nonstop.

DUMBBELL ROMANIAN DEADLIFT

Great for:
track and field, wrestling

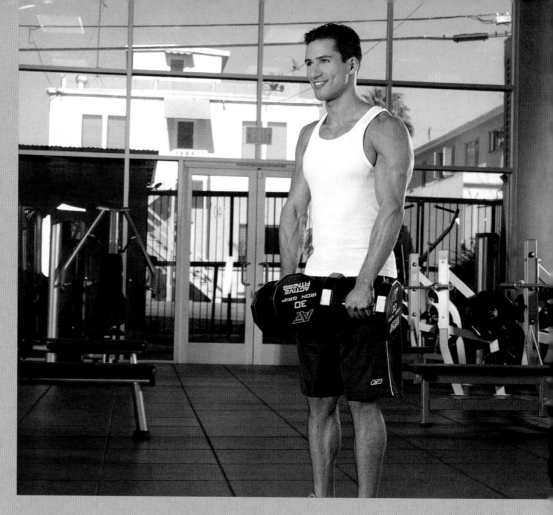

Get ready!

Hold a dumbbell in each hand in front of your thighs.

Go!

With a slight lower-back arch, push your butt back while bending forward at the hips. Lower your torso until the weights are at the middle of your shins. Push back up to the starting position. Keep your back slightly arched throughout.

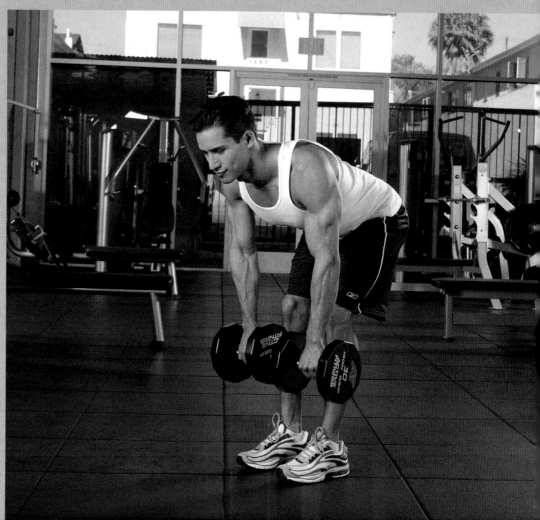

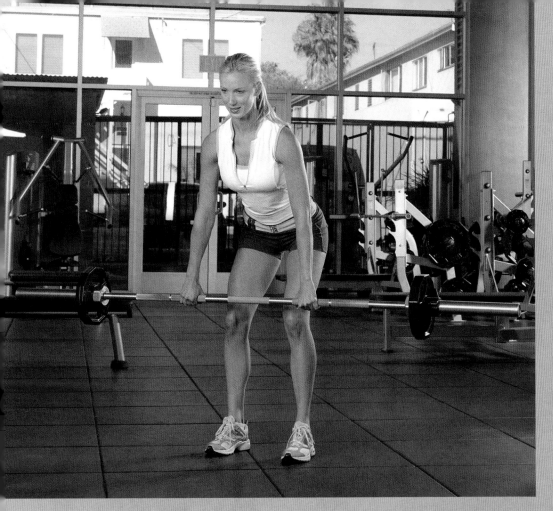

BENT-OVER BARBELL ROW

Great for:
volleyball, bowling

Get ready!
Stand holding a barbell with an overhand grip, hands spaced slightly wider than shoulder-width apart, feet shoulder-width apart, knees bent slightly. Bend forward at the waist to angle forward your torso.

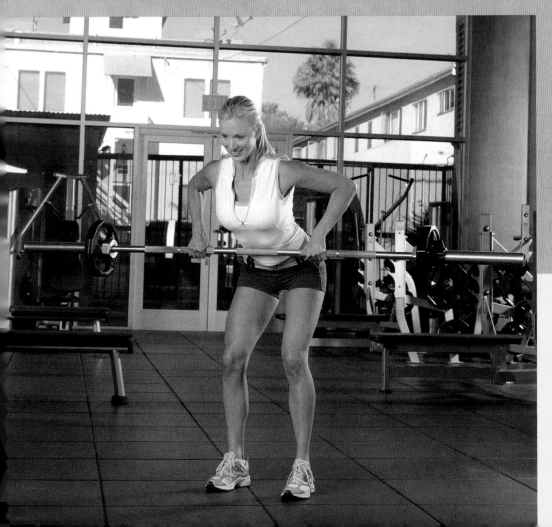

Go!
Draw the bar toward your rib cage, so that your elbows come straight back. Pause for a split second and then lower the barbell back down.

Watch out for:
Rounding your back. That usually means you're going too heavy.

107

SQUAT THRUST

Great for:
volleyball,
football

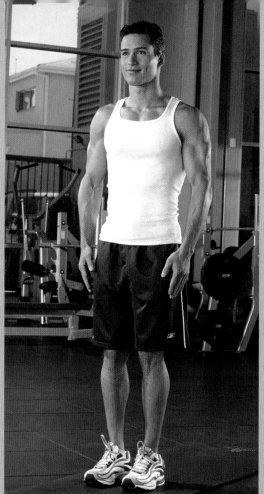

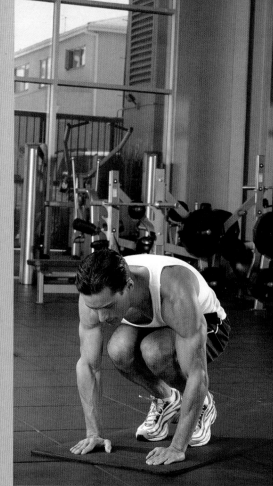

Get ready!

Stand with your feet shoulder-width apart.

Go!

Bend at the hips and knees to lower your body as far as you can, as if you were squatting. Only instead of coming back up, place your hands on the floor and straighten your legs behind you to assume a pushup position. Perform a pushup, then draw your knees back toward your chest until your feet are beneath you. Stand up to return to the starting position.

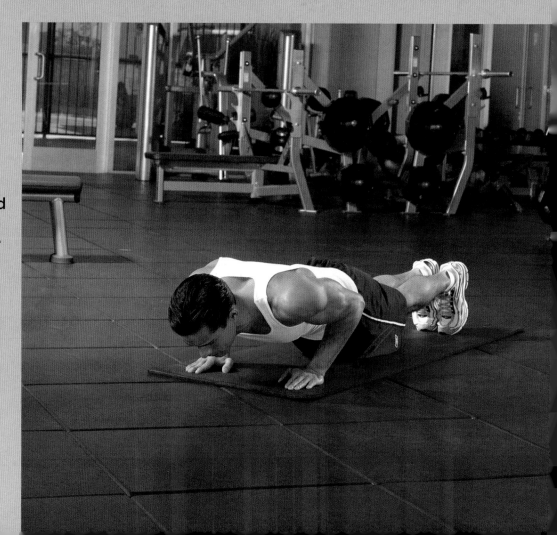

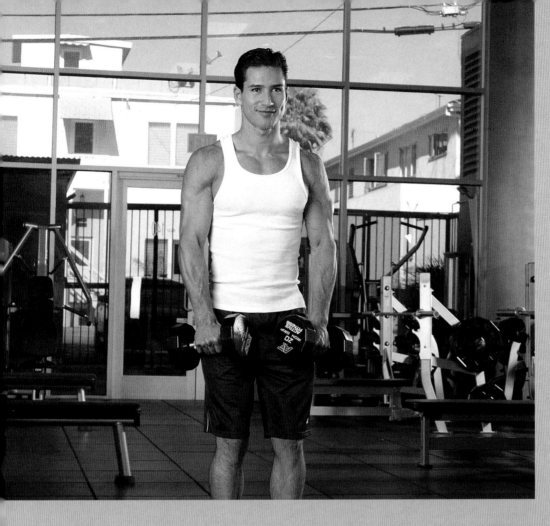

DUMBBELL LATERAL RAISE

Great for: boxing, baseball

Get ready!

Hold a light dumbbell in each hand, arms at your sides. Plant your feet hip-width apart. Bend your knees slightly.

Go!

Keeping your arms straight, elbows unlocked, slowly sweep your arms out to the sides until they're parallel to the floor, at which point your palms should face down and your body should resemble the letter T. Slowly lower your arms back down to your sides.

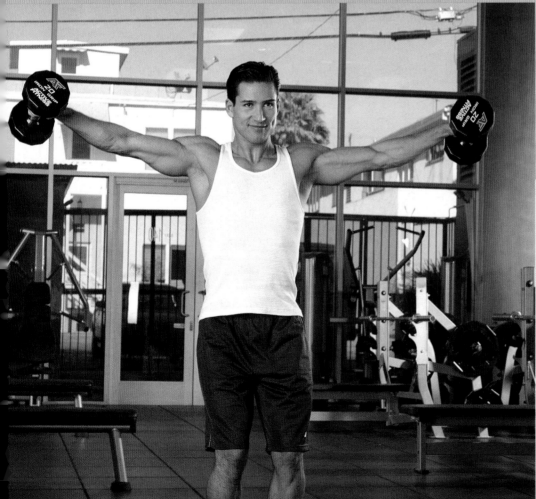

Watch out for:

The delicate architecture of your shoulder joints. Never cheat by swinging the weights up on this move—you're inviting injury. In fact, it doesn't hurt to do this move, especially the lowering part, almost in slow motion.

LYING DUMBBELL TRICEPS EXTENSION

Great for: baseball, basketball

Get ready!

Lie face-up on a flat bench with your knees bent and your feet near the end of the bench. Hold two light dumbbells overhead, arms fully extended, palms facing each other in a neutral grip. Your arms should resemble goal posts.

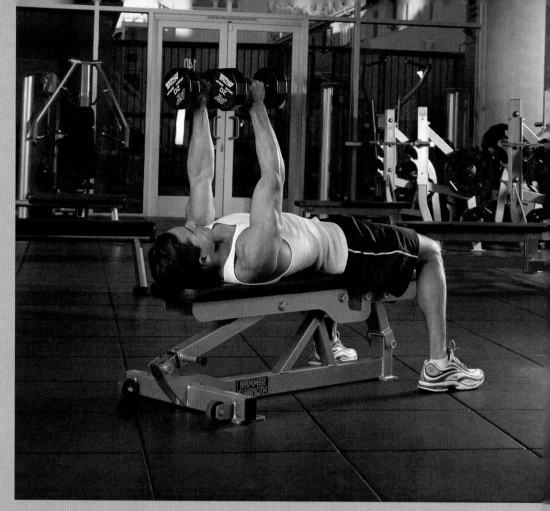

Go!

Bend your elbows to lower the weights until they're six inches or so from your face. Extend your elbows to slowly push the weights back up.

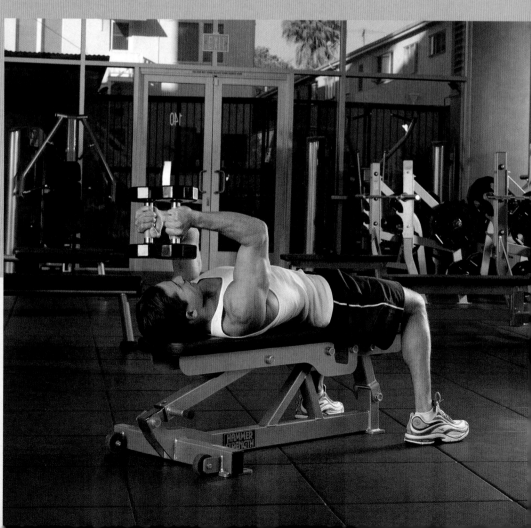

Watch out for:

Excessive movement in your upper arms. Those should remain more or less fixed as you bend your elbow. Also, watch your head!

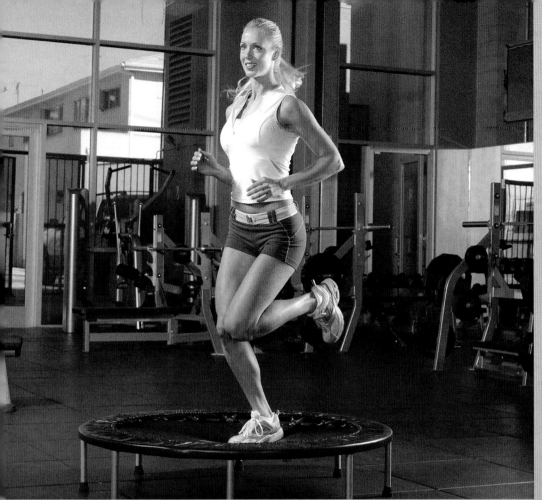

MINI-TRAMPOLINE JOGGING

Great for:
boxing, dance

Get ready!
Stand on a mini-trampoline.

Go!
Jog, kicking your knees nice and high.

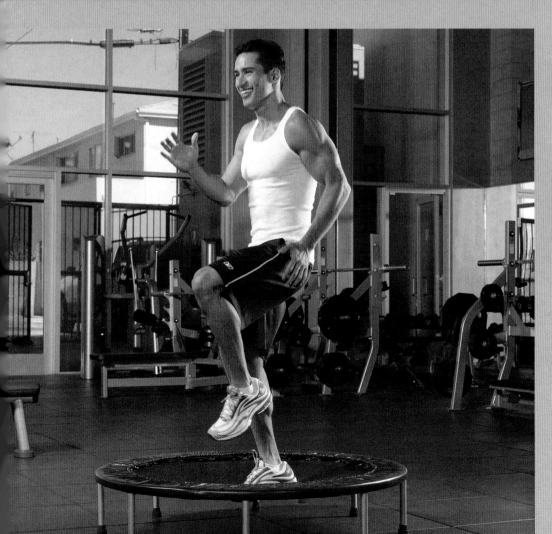

111

CABLE REVERSE WOOD CHOP

Great for: boxing, discus throw

Get ready!

Attach a rope handle to a low pulley. Stand perpendicular to the cable stack. Bend at the waist and knees. Rotate your torso toward the stack and grasp the handle with both hands.

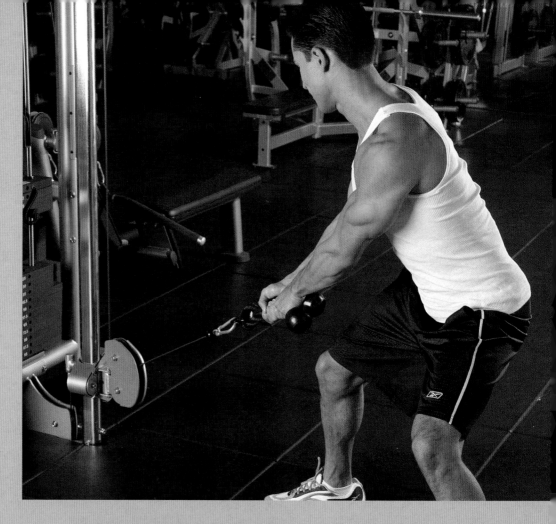

Go!

Without changing a slight bend in your elbows, explosively rotate your torso in the other direction, and up, to execute the move. By the time the handle has traveled across your body, you should be upright. Return to the starting position. After completing your reps, reverse your body position and do the same number.

Watch out for:

Swinging with your arms only. The idea is to work the core by rotating your torso. Your arms are just along for the ride.

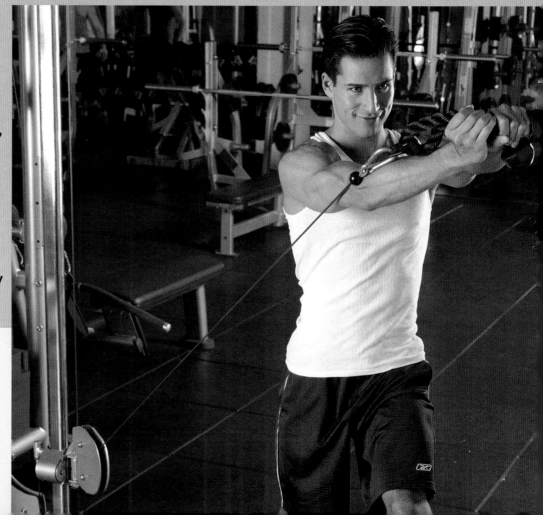

10-MINUTE WORKOUT TOTAL-BODY CIRCUIT

You'll need a gym to complete this full-body workout, but it's well worth the effort. In fact, this is one of the most efficient training sessions you'll ever encounter.

Exercise	Sets	Reps	Rest (seconds)
Front squat (See page 189 for exercise description.)	3	10–12	Up to 15
Flat-bench barbell press (See page 182 for exercise description.)	3	10–12	Up to 15
Dumbbell Romanian deadlift (See page 106 for exercise description.)	3	10–12	Up to 15
Horizontal pullup (Lie under the racked bar of a Smith machine holding the bar so that your arms are straight and your legs extend straight out before you. Pull your chest up to the bar and then return to the starting position.	3	10–12	Up to 15
Seated dumbbell curl/shoulder press (See page 30 for exercise description.)	3	10–12	Up to 15
Reverse crunch (See page 32 for exercise description.)	3	10–12	Up to 120

6 SIGNS YOU WORK OUT TOO MUCH (OR TOO HARD)

1) You lose weight too quickly. As a general rule, you don't want to lose more than two pounds per week. Exception: As you build more muscle, you'll shed fat more easily, so you might shed three or even four pounds for a few weeks. Anything more than that, however, is a sign that you're probably not eating enough to fuel your new muscle, which will shrink without proper protein feedings.

2) You spontaneously add sets and reps. No one ever got anywhere in the gym without pushing the envelope, but for the most part, your progress should be a function of meticulous planning, not a spur-of-the-moment thing. The more time you spend in the gym, the easier it might seem to tack on a few more exercises. It might work for a few days, but you could eventually burn out by doing this and wind up missing workouts. In short: Stick with a plan like the one you're holding in your hands.

3) You suffer a nagging injury . . . and another . . . and another. You're working in part to become as healthy as possible. If you're working out so much that you're chronically icing down the pain of bursitis, tendonitis, or achy joints, then your workouts have become counterproductive. If you strike the right balance, the gym will energize your entire day, not land you in the trainer's room.

4) You've hit a plateau. Strength and size don't increase ad infinitum. As your body adapts to increased workloads, the pace of your gains will slow. The normal remedy for this is to vary your approach or hit the gym harder, but if you've stayed on a plateau for more than two weeks, chances are you're working *too* hard. Back off. Recover.

5) Your appetite is decreasing. The right combination of diet and exercise will put your body in an anabolic (i.e., muscle growth) state, meaning you're going to be hungry nearly all the time. Overworking your muscles, however, will stifle your appetite, sending your body into catabolic (the opposite of anabolic) panic. It's a surefire way to lose your hard-earned muscle.

6) You're not invited to your own slumber party. It's a common problem afflicting many serious athletes: They burn calories all day with a rigorous exercise program, only to find that their well-deserved sleep eludes them. This is usually the result of over-stimulated muscles that work so often they can't stop firing even when you lie down.

Phase II:
Workout B Weights and Cardio

Sequence	Week	Exercise	Sets[1]	Reps[2]	Rest[3]
A1	1	Dumbbell Step-up	3	10–12/leg	↓
	2	Dumbbell Step-up	3	10–12/leg	↓
	3	Dumbbell Step-up	3	10–12/leg	↓
	4	Dumbbell Step-up	3	10–12/leg	↓
A2	1	Incline Bench Dumbbell Press	3	10–12	↓
	2	Incline Bench Dumbbell Press	3	10–12	↓
	3	Incline Bench Dumbbell Press	3	10–12	↓
	4	Incline Bench Dumbbell Press	3	10–12	↓
A3	1	Skipping Rope	3	1 minute	60
	2	Skipping Rope	3	1 minute	60
	3	Skipping Rope	3	1 minute	60
	4	Skipping Rope	3	1 minute	60
B1	1	Swiss Ball Leg Curl	3	10–12	↓
	2	Swiss Ball Leg Curl	3	10–12	↓
	3	Swiss Ball Leg Curl	3	10–12	↓
	4	Swiss Ball Leg Curl	3	10–12	↓
B2	1	Seated Rope Handle Cable Row	3	10–12	↓
	2	Seated Rope Handle Cable Row	3	10–12	↓
	3	Seated Rope Handle Cable Row	3	10–12	↓
	4	Seated Rope Handle Cable Row	3	10–12	↓
B3	1	Mountain Climber	3	15–25	60
	2	Mountain Climber	3	15–25	60
	3	Mountain Climber	3	15–25	60
	4	Mountain Climber	3	15–25	60
C1	1	Standing Alternating Dumbbell Shoulder Press	3	10–12	↓
	2	Standing Alternating Dumbbell Shoulder Press	3	10–12	↓
	3	Standing Alternating Dumbbell Shoulder Press	3	10–12	↓
	4	Standing Alternating Dumbbell Shoulder Press	3	10–12	↓
C2	1	E-Z Bar Curl	3	10–12	↓
	2	E-Z Bar Curl	3	10–12	↓
	3	E-Z Bar Curl	3	10–12	↓
	4	E-Z Bar Curl	3	10–12	↓
C3	1	Soccer Touch Drill	3	Up to 45 seconds	60
	2	Soccer Touch Drill	3	Up to 45 seconds	60
	3	Soccer Touch Drill	3	Up to 45 seconds	60
	4	Soccer Touch Drill	3	Up to 45 seconds	60
D1	1	Standing Cable Chop	3	10–12/side	60
	2	Standing Cable Chop	3	10–12/side	60
	3	Standing Cable Chop	3	10–12/side	60
	4	Standing Cable Chop	3	10–12/side	60
E1		Perform rowing intervals: Row for 3 minutes at a easy pace, then perform 6–8 repetitions of 30–60 seconds each, followed by 90–120 seconds of rest.			

[1] Do modified supersets with each pair of exercises listed with the same number (for example, A1 and A2); that is, do the prescribed number of sets for each of the two exercises in alternating fashion before moving on to the next pairing. (For example, if the program calls for three sets, do one set of split squats followed by one set of push-ups, and then repeat twice). Rest in between each set as prescribed.

[2] The last rep you can finish with complete control and perfect form should fall within this range, so select your weight accordingly. Once you have completed all your repetitions with your current weight for two consecutive workouts, increase your poundage slightly. Five pounds for each new step is a good rule of thumb.

[3] Between supersets, measured in seconds.

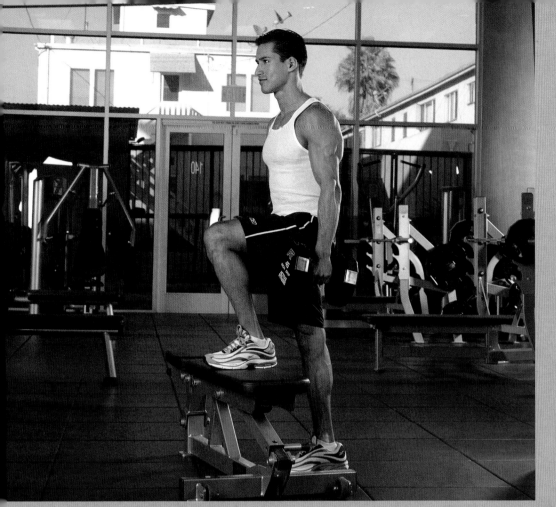

DUMBBELL STEP-UP

Great for: mountain climbing, sprinting

Get ready!

Holding a dumbbell in each hand, stand before a bench or box just tall enough that your thighs become parallel with the floor when you step onto its surface.

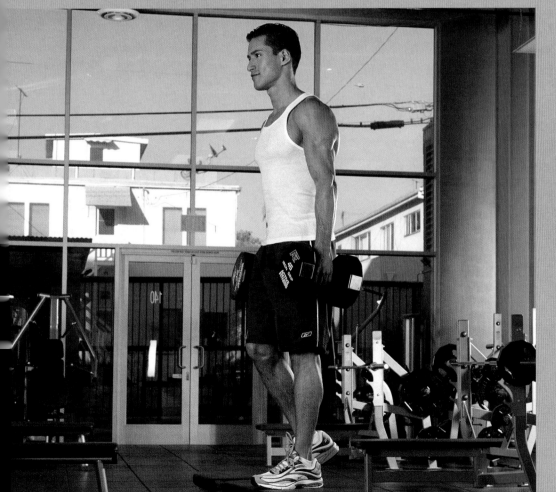

Go!

Lift one foot and place it on the raised surface and, without hesitation, push your body up until your weight-bearing leg is straight and your other foot trails away from the bench. Return to the starting position.

INCLINE BENCH DUMBBELL PRESS

Great for: football, volleyball

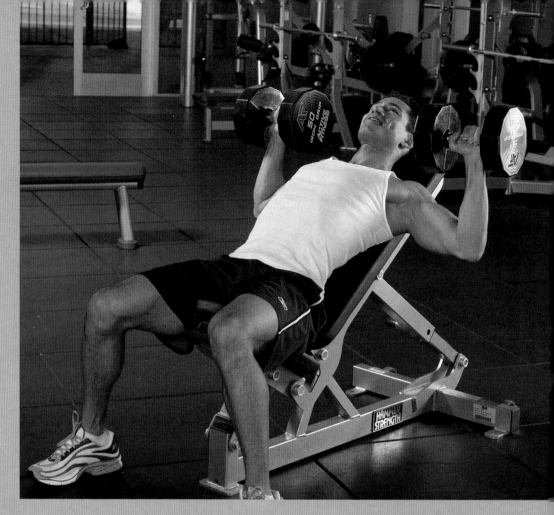

Get ready!

Lie facing up on a bench set at a 30- to 45-degree angle. Hold a pair of dumbbells outside your chest with an overhand grip, palms facing forward.

Go!

Press the weights straight above your chest. They should arc close together, yet not touch. After a moment's pause, lower them to the starting position.

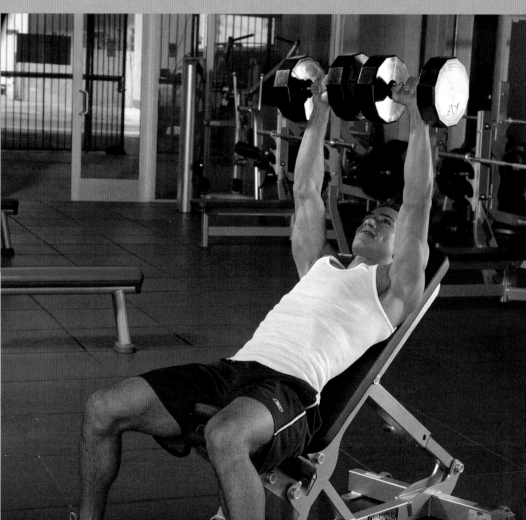

Watch out for:

Excessive bend of the wrists. Try to keep them straight throughout the exercise.

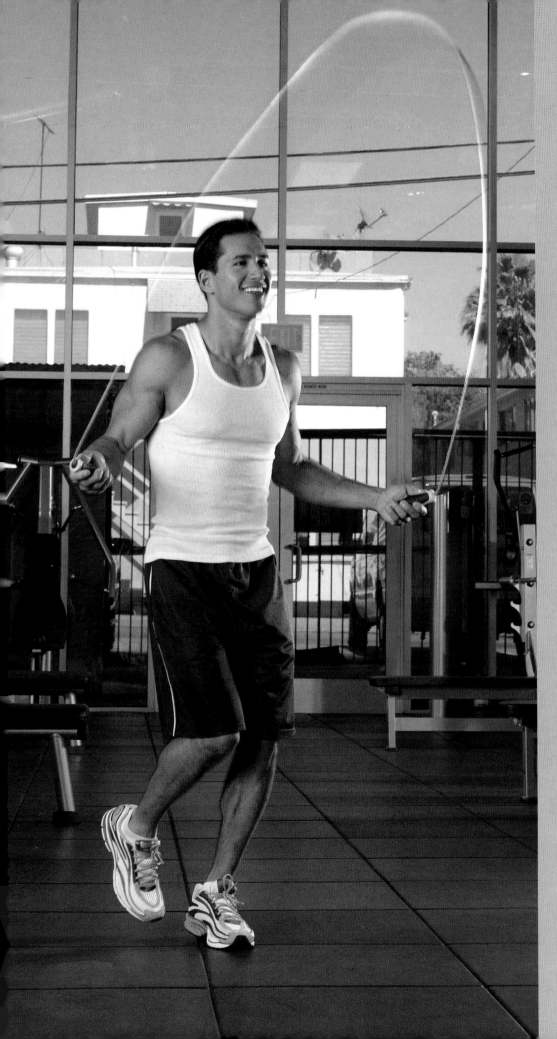

SKIPPING ROPE

Great for: boxing, dance

Get ready!
Stand holding a jump rope.

Go!
Jump!

SWISS BALL LEG CURL

Great for:
swimming, soccer

Get ready!

Lie on your back on the floor with your lower legs and ankles elevated on a Swiss ball, so that your heels are perched on top. Your arms should be positioned alongside your torso; this will help you stay balanced. Raise your hips so that your body forms a straight line.

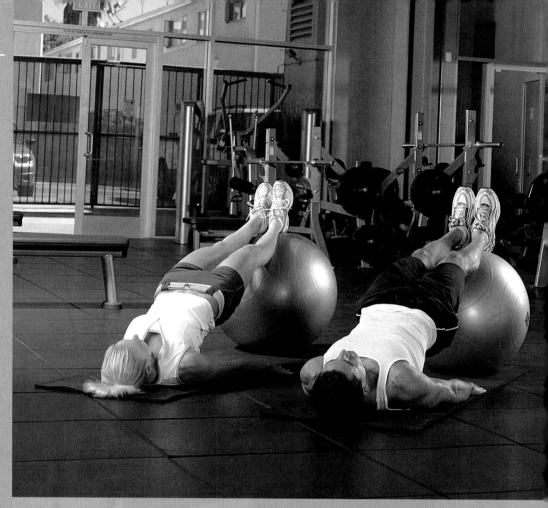

Go!

Squeezing your butt, use your heels to drag the ball toward you. Your knees should reach 90 degrees at full contraction. Roll the ball back to the starting position using your heels.

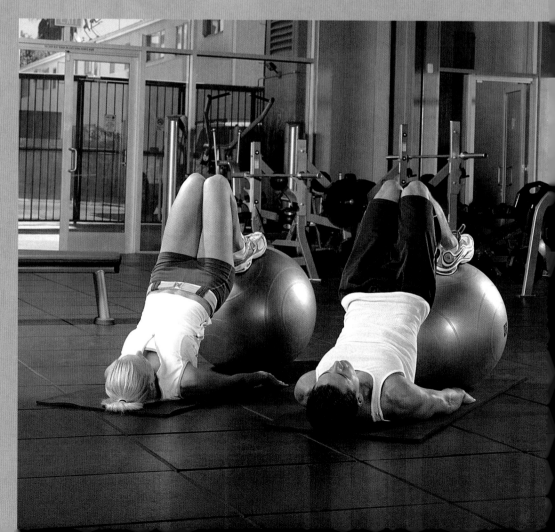

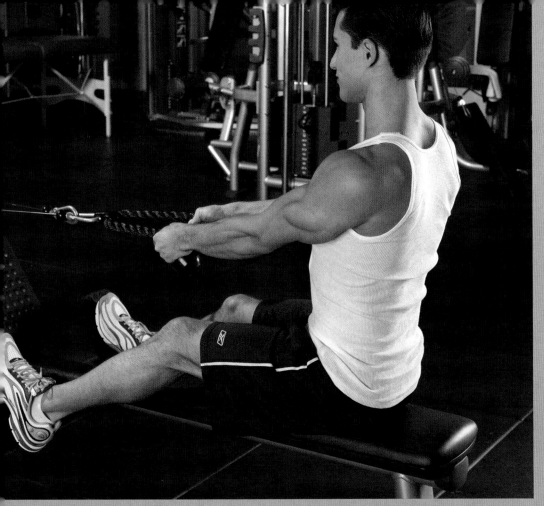

SEATED ROPE-HANDLE CABLE ROW

Great for:
tug of war,
hammer throw

Get ready!

Attach a split rope handle to a seated row machine. Bend forward to grab the two strands of rope so that your palms face each other.

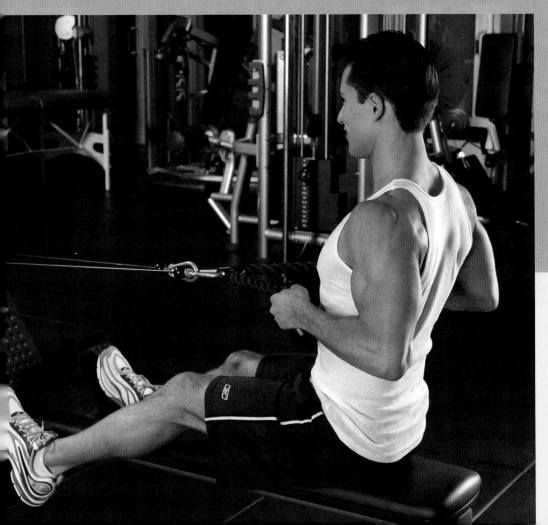

Go!

Keeping your back straight, squeeze back your shoulder blades. Pulling with your elbows, not your hands, draw the handle in toward your midsection, then slowly straighten your arms back out in front of you.

Watch out for:

Excessive forward leaning on the negative half of the rep. Let your arms carry the handle back; don't lunge forward by bending excessively at the hips.

119

MOUNTAIN CLIMBER

Great for:
football, rugby

Get ready!

Assume the standard pushup position: (A) hands on the floor in line with your shoulders, but hands spaced slightly wider than shoulder-width apart; and (B) legs straightened behind you. Your body should resemble a plank from head to heels.

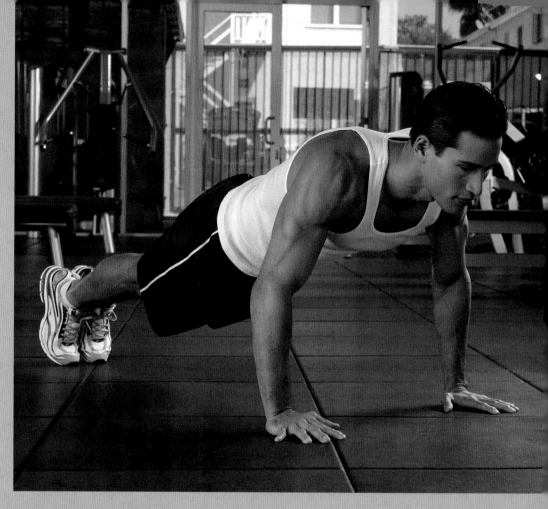

Go!

Bring your left knee toward your chest on the same side, and without hesitating, bring your right leg forward while extending your left leg back.

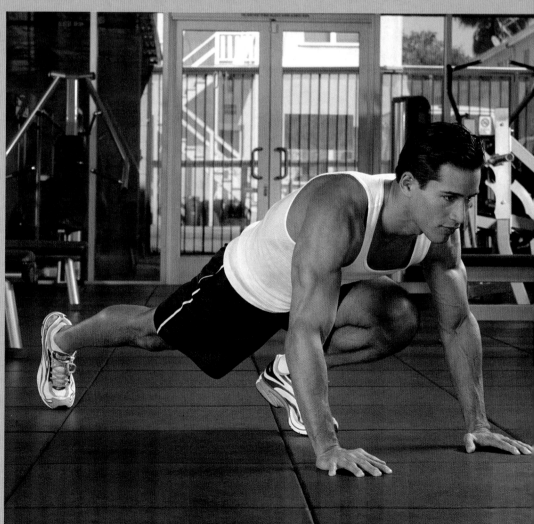

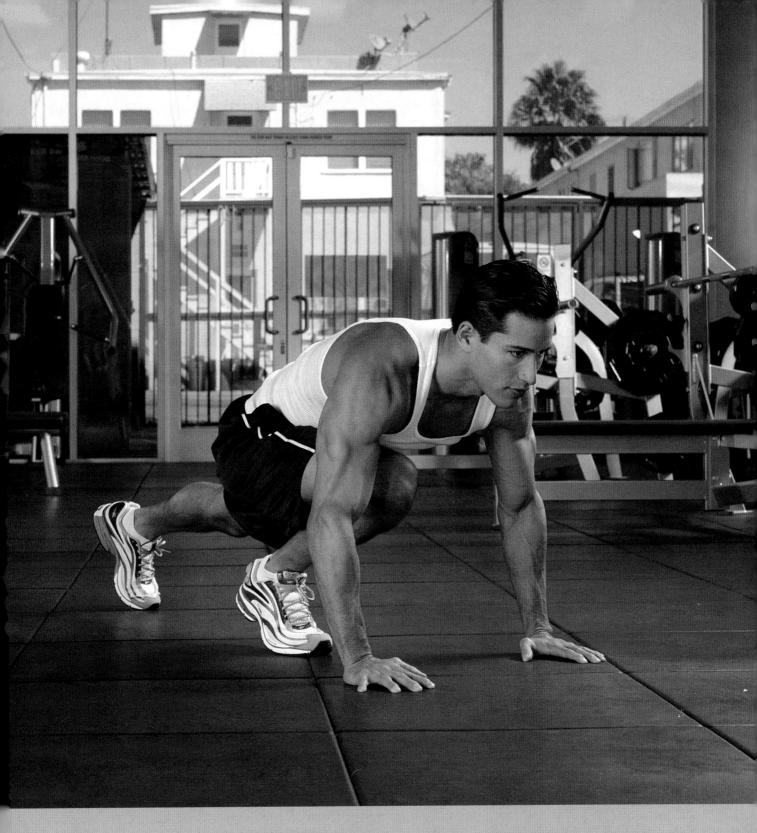

Continue in alternating fashion, "running" like a sprinter on the floor.

STANDING ALTERNATING DUMBBELL SHOULDER PRESS

Great for:
boxing, archery

Get ready!

Stand holding a dumbbell in each hand just above and outside of your shoulders, palms facing forward.

Go!

Drive one weight straight above you, until your arm is fully extended. Slowly lower the dumbbell back to the starting position. Repeat using the other arm. Continue alternating until you've completed all reps.

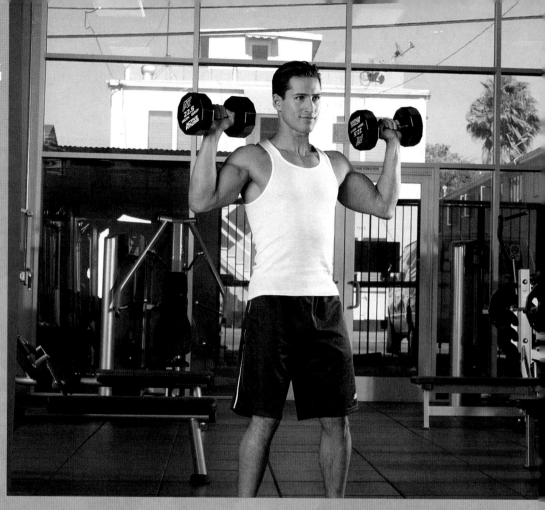

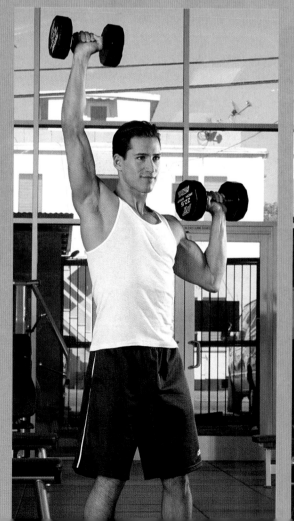

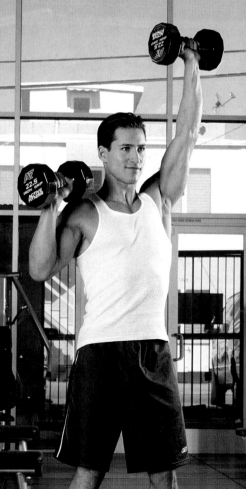

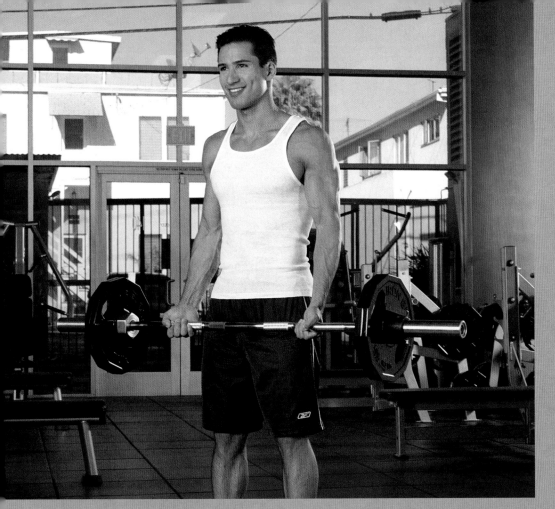

E-Z BAR CURL

Great for: football, rugby

Get ready!

Stand holding a loaded EZ-bar with an underhand grip—hands shoulder-width apart—at arm's length, so that your hands nearly touch your thighs.

Go!

Curl the bar up to the front of your shoulders, squeezing your biceps hard at the top. Lower it back down.

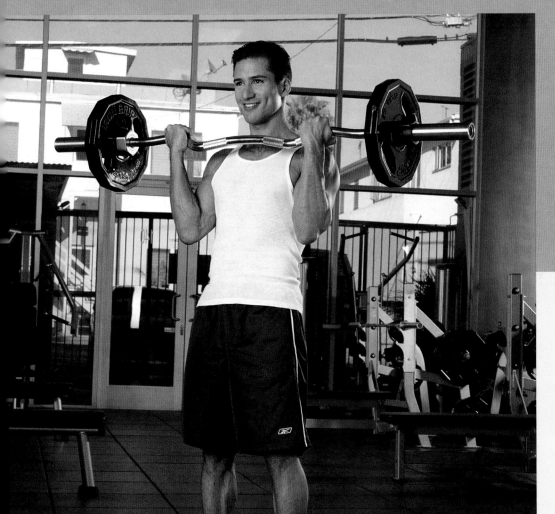

Watch out for:

Excessive arm movement. Throughout the entire rep, keep your upper arms pinned against your sides. Your elbows should function like hinges.

123

SOCCER TOUCH DRILL

Great for:
soccer,
basketball

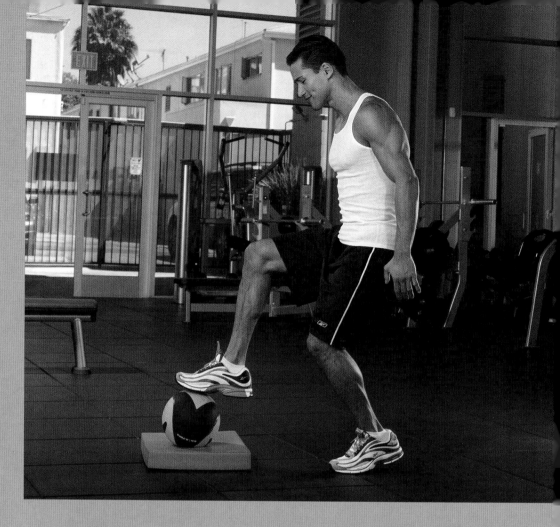

Get ready!

Place a medicine ball on a foam pad in front of you.

Go!

Gently place one foot on top of the ball; then begin quickly changing feet rapidly. Continue without knocking the medicine ball off its support.

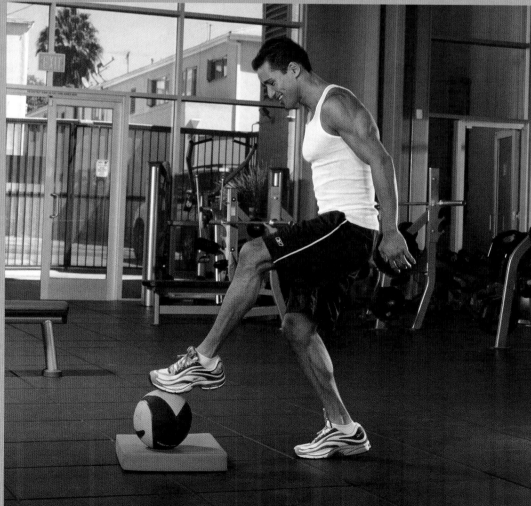

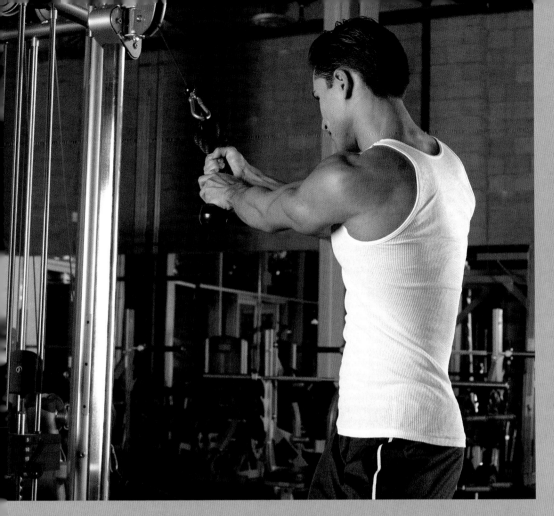

STANDING CABLE CHOP

Great for: martial arts, lacrosse

Get ready!

Attach a rope handle to a high pulley. Stand perpendicular to the cable stack. Rotate your torso toward the stack and grasp the handle with both hands to assume the starting position.

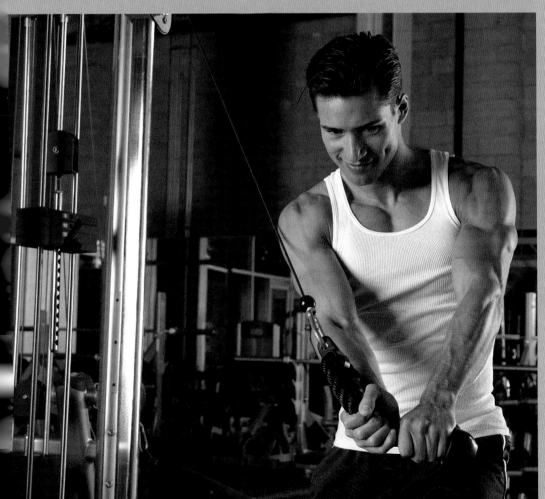

Go!

With a slight bend in your elbows, explosively rotate your torso in the other direction, and down, to execute the move. Return to the starting position. After completing your reps, reverse your body position and do the same number.

Phase II:
Workout C: Yoga
SHIFTING SHAPES:
MY FLEXIBILITY WORKOUT

I love hitting the weight room and training like Arnold did. I love doing interval sprints, too. And boxing is probably my greatest passion when it comes to physical fitness.

Flexibility training didn't come as naturally to me as those other activities did. Yet I've come to realize that it's equally important. Never did I realize that more acutely than when I performed on *Dancing with the Stars*. The most demanding dances were all the ballroom dances. I was amazed how much holding those frames stretched out my back muscles in particular. That was quite a workout because my muscles weren't used to it. Salsa and mambo were a little less taxing—I just felt like I was having a good time.

That flexibility training helps with injury prevention goes without saying. Tight, inelastic muscle tissue is highly prone to pulling and tearing when it suddenly needs to move, a tendency that only increases as you age. I'm not just talking about the weekend warrior who goes out and pulls a hammie in right field during a softball game, either. Don't become one of those people who slip on an icy driveway and feel an underused back muscle pop.

What I've learned over time is that flexibility also plays a huge role in performance in the gym, on the field, or on the court. Ever wonder why a guy the size of Tiger Woods can hit drives like cannon shots? Flexibility. Wonder why a relatively small guy like Jake Peavy can wind up and throw a baseball that travels 95 miles per hour? Flexibility. The same goes for Andy Roddick and his blazing serve, not to mention virtually every other elite athlete, including boxers. It's Physics 101: the longer the lever arm, the more time to generate force.

I love subjecting my body to different workout forms, but yoga is among my favorites. I usually do it on Sundays. I'll get up early, go for a run, come back, have a little breakfast, and then go to yoga. I really like it, and I love the chilled, Zen feeling that follows a yoga session.

I don't profess to be an expert at yoga, so I worked closely with a top expert, Kimberly Snyder, to compile the following sequence of moves in this book. Kimberly began studying yoga in the Himalayan Mountains and was trained and certified by the great yogi master Sri Dharma Mittra, with whom she continues to be an avid student. She also teaches group classes for various health clubs.

Yoga for Flexibility

Do this routine once a week during Phase II, on days when you're not lifting or interval training. Feel free to use any of the moves listed as post-workout stretches, too, or after work, when you wake up. Heck, you really can't become too limber.

Instructions:

● Move from pose to pose in the order given.

● Breathe through your nose, always trying to draw the air down into your belly. Never hold your breath in any pose.

● Think of this as a natural and slow progression in which the body begins to "open up." For many of these poses, "advancing" means *going deeper.* In yoga, quality is more important than quantity. That's why many of the counts are similar for beginners and the advanced alike.

HEY, MARIO!

I'm spending a lot of time on the beach. Can any supplement help prevent skin cancer?

Immune-boosting vitamin D is a great overall cancer fighter, skin cancer included. A recent study in the *American Journal of Clinical Nutrition* found that women who supplemented daily with 1,000 international units of vitamin D experienced 60 to 77 percent fewer cancer incidences over a four-year span than women in a placebo group. Scientists believe the same benefits apply to guys.

DOWNWARD DOG

Spread both palms out on the floor, with all 10 fingers pressing firmly into the floor. Now step back with both legs so that your arms and legs are straight, and your body forms a V. Lift your hips as high as possible, and gently press your heels down without bending your knees. Your feet should be parallel, hip distance or so apart; and your head should be relaxed between your arms. *Stay in this pose for 3 to 5 breaths.*

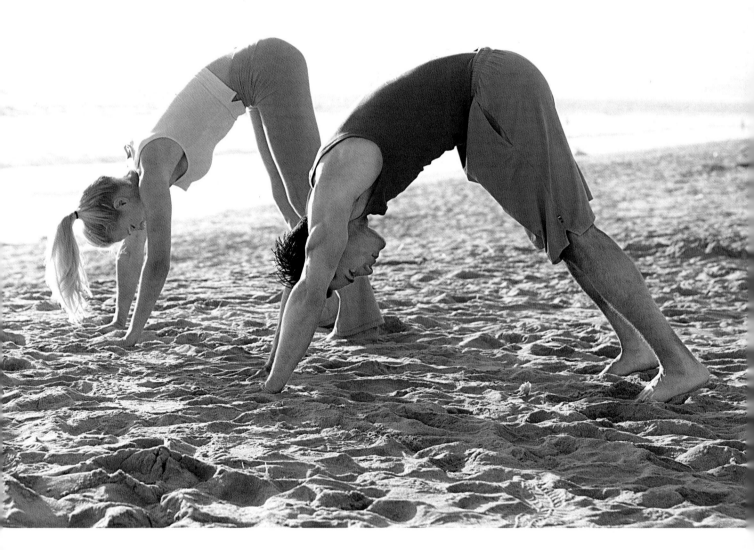

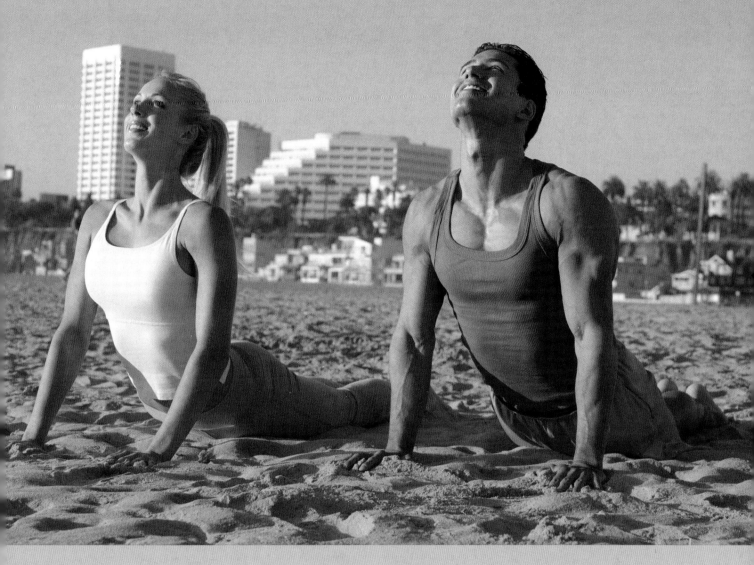

UPWARD DOG

Lie on the floor on your stomach. Your feet should be about a foot apart, toes pointed straight back. Place your palms on the floor near either side of your chest. As your inhale, raise your head and trunk and stretch your arms to a completely straight position, then push your head and trunk back as far as possible. Your legs should remain straight and tightened at the knees, which should be pushed off the ground. Your body weight should rest on your palms and tops of your feet. *Stay in this pose for 2 to 3 breaths. This completes one sequence. Start with 1 to 2 sequences and progress up 5. Depending on your starting point, this could take a few weeks to several months.*

SEATED FORWARD BEND

Sit on the floor with your legs stretched in front of you, big toes touching, feet flexed. Stretch both arms over your head with an inhalation; on the next exhalation, stretch both arms in front, parallel to your legs. Your hands can catch hold of your toes or feet, or your palms can rest on the ground. If you're insufficiently flexible to perform the move as described, bend your knees to where your chest and thighs are touching, then gradually try to straighten your legs inch by inch over time. *Stay in this pose for 5 to 15 breaths. This completes 1 sequence. As your body starts to "open up" over time, it will bend farther.*

SEATED FORWARD FOLD WITH BENT LEG

Sit on the floor with your legs stretched out in front of you. Bend your left knee and move your left foot into the inside of your right thigh. On the inhalation, raise and straighten your arms over your head, and twist your body so that your torso is facing your right foot. On the next exhalation, stretch down and forward, toward your right foot. You can hold on to your foot, catch your hands around your foot, or place your palms on the ground. (Beginners can place a towel around their foot and, holding on with two hands, gently pull their torso down and forward.) Repeat with your left foot stretched out and your right foot bent in. *Hold each side for 3 to 5 breaths. Going to each side completes 1 sequence. Progress by going deeper over time.*

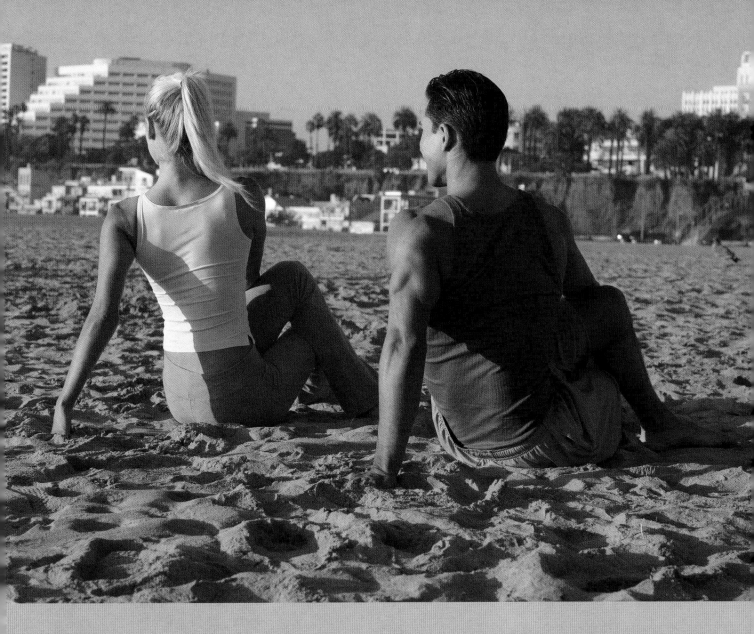

SEATED SPINAL TWIST

Sit on the floor with both legs straight out in front of you. Bend your left leg over your right leg, letting the sole of your left foot rest either above or below the knee joint. Pressing your left palm on the ground close to your spine, inhale as your lift your right arm up, and then tuck your right elbow across the outside of your right knee. Your right arm should remain vertical as your body twists 90 degrees to the left. *Follow the same instructions given for seated forward fold with bent leg.*

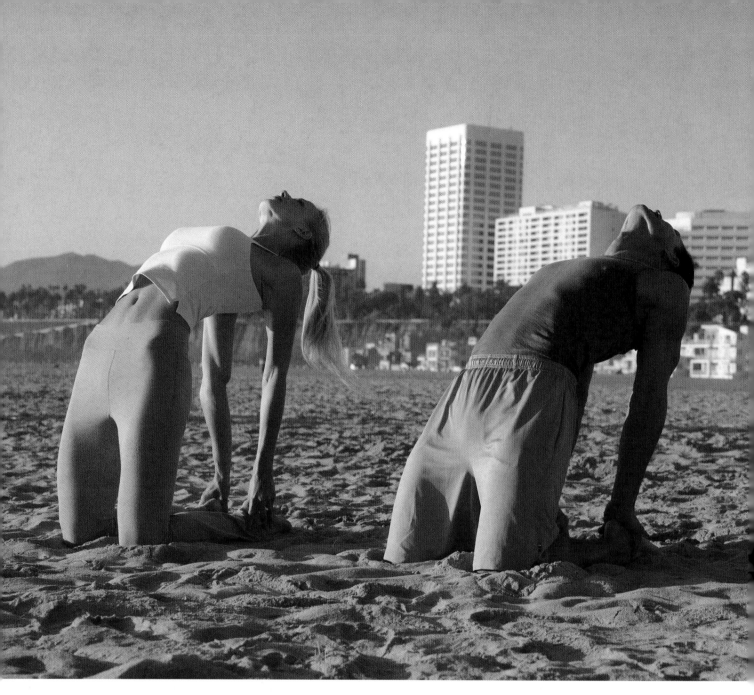

CAMEL

Kneel on the floor, keeping your knees and feet about hip-distance apart, with the tops of your feet pressing into the floor and your toes pointing away from your body. Rest your palms on your hips with your thumbs facing up. On the inhalation, start to curve back your spine and head, while extending your ribs and pressing your pelvis and thighs forward. You may rest your hands on the floor behind you for support. When you're ready to come up, inhale and make your spine vertical again. *Hold for 3 to 5 breaths. Repeat 3 times. Over time, the back bend should become deeper.*

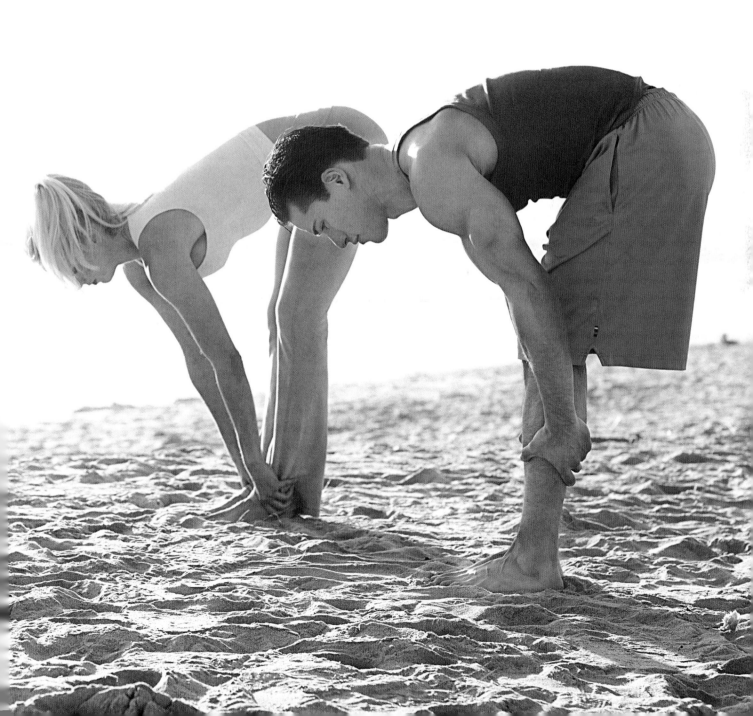

Phase II:
Workout D: Basketball

PUMPED:
MY BASKETBALL
WORKOUTS

Basketball may be the one sport that can give boxing a run for its money as far as physical demands go. To excel, all you have to do is run fast, jump through the roof, muscle past defenders, cut on a dime, outmaneuver ball-hawking defenders who come at you like video game attackers, and then shoot an orange sphere through an 18-inch hoop raised 10 feet off the ground. What could be easier than that, right?

Kobe and LeBron don't have to be worried, but I'm a seriously dedicated recreational hoopster. I used to play in something called the NBA Entertainment League, which was an L.A.-based league at Crossroads High School in Santa Monica. Many actors and musical artists would lace 'em up, and we had refs, jerseys—the whole nine yards. I played with or against Ice Cube, Brian McKnight, Dean Cain, Jaleel White, and a bunch of hip-hop guys.

Luckily, I'm not asking you to excel. I'm asking you to play and practice in order to break a sweat. This book is about shaping up, not trying out for the Lakers. If you've actually got game, consider it a bonus.

Throughout this book, interval training reigns supreme. Lo and behold, here's a sport consisting entirely of stops and starts, punctuated by shots and jumps (and some occasional trash talk). That's why intense interval training is better for basketball than running along the side of the road at the same pace for five miles. That's as boring as it sounds—whereas with basketball drills, at least you're having fun, even as you get totally wiped out. Women shouldn't hesitate to try it, either. Throw on a headband, tie you hair in a pony tail, and rock it. It's an unbelievably enjoyable game for everyone. If you are shy about playing with a group of guys, just let them know you want to give it a try or ask a group of friends to play. Everyone has played basketball at some point in their lives and you can encourage them to rekindle their enjoyment of this game. Don't forget that you can always find a hoop and do some shooting on your own. Just remember to keep moving and dribbling as you move from shot to shot.

The moves you're doing in the gym are precisely what it takes to improve your basketball game—just as playing basketball will elevate your cardiovascular fitness to new heights. Balanced development is important, but hips and legs are particularly important in hoops. The dumbbell squat, a key move in Phase II, is the classic exercise for working these muscle groups. But you also need speed, agility, and explosiveness, which I help you develop with exercises such as bench jumps and medicine ball throws.

Since San Diego, my hometown, doesn't have a basketball team, the Lakers are my team. I live only ten minutes from the Staples Center, where they play in Los Angeles. But if you watch any NBA or NCAA basketball teams train, you'll see them doing straight sprints one day, change-of-direction sprints the next, and then on another day, running in a pool. You may not be ready to take that training plunge, but you have to at least give this workout a try, because it's one of my all-time favorites. Basically, I've taken several of my favorite conditioning drills and arranged them into one bad-to-the-bone cardio workout. In Phase II, you have the option of doing this once a week, on a day when you're not in the gym. (Of course, I have to add the usual disclaimer: WORKING OUT MORE THAN RECOMMENDED CAN LEAD TO OVERTRAINING. If you do this workout, eliminate one of your post-workout interval sessions that same week.

One caveat when you're playing basketball, as opposed to training for it: More than any other activity discussed in this book—except for perhaps boxing—basketball places your body at risk of injury. If you're playing four-on-four or five-on-five—or even just horsing around one-on-one style with a friend at the local court—you're talking about bodies jumping, cutting, and colliding within a comparatively small area under the basket. Injuries can range from sprained ankles and jammed fingers—both are almost a given in this sport—to something as devastating as a torn anterior cruciate ligament, which can require reconstructive knee surgery and lay you up for months. To lessen the risk of injury, *always* play within your physical limitations.

Those of you suiting it up for the first time ever:

- Run 400 meters—a little less than four football field lengths—at three-quarters speed. Rest 3 minutes. Repeat this run/rest sequence 3 times, for 4 sets total.

- Progress over time to where you're running 200 meters—a little less than two football field lengths—8 times, resting 1 minute in between; and then 100 meters 8 times, resting 30 seconds in between.

Those of you who've played some organized ball:

1) 5 and a halfs. Sprint to one baseline and back 5 times. On the sixth, stop at half court.

2) Sidewinders. Run back and forth between sidelines (not baselines) for 60 seconds.

3) Suicides. You did these in high school, right? Run hard from a baseline to the near foul line and back, to midcourt and back, to the far foul line and back, and then to the far baseline and back.

4) Reverse suicides. Do the same thing as above, only go longest increment to shortest instead.

Progress to where you can perform 2 to 4 sets of all four drills, resting 1 minute in between.

Phase II, Workout D alternate: Raquetball

If I can't make it to the basketball court that day, there's a good chance you'll find me playing racquetball. Not only is this game a great workout, it produces rivers of sweat if played correctly—and it's also amazing for developing hand-eye coordination. So feel free to substitute my racquetball workout for my basketball workout.

FOUR-CORNERS DRILL

Beginners

Place the ball in the middle of the court. Stand in one corner. Run to the center, grab the ball, sprint back to the same corner, and then sprint back to center to place where it started. Run to the next corner and repeat the sequence. Repeat for all corners.

Intermediate and Advanced

Place the ball in the middle of the court. Stand in one corner. Run to the center and grab the ball, sprint back to the other corner on the same side, immediately sprint to the opposite corner and back, then return the ball to center. Repeat from all four corners.

LATERAL POWER SHUFFLE

Stand in the middle of the back wall. Leap forward off one foot as far as possible. Immediately shuffle to one side of the court and touch the wall. Immediately shuffle back to the center. Shuffle backward to the starting position. Repeat the leap forward, but this time shuffle to the opposite wall. Each time you've touched both sides and run backwards, double the number of initial leaps. The drill ends when you reach the front wall with your forward leaps.

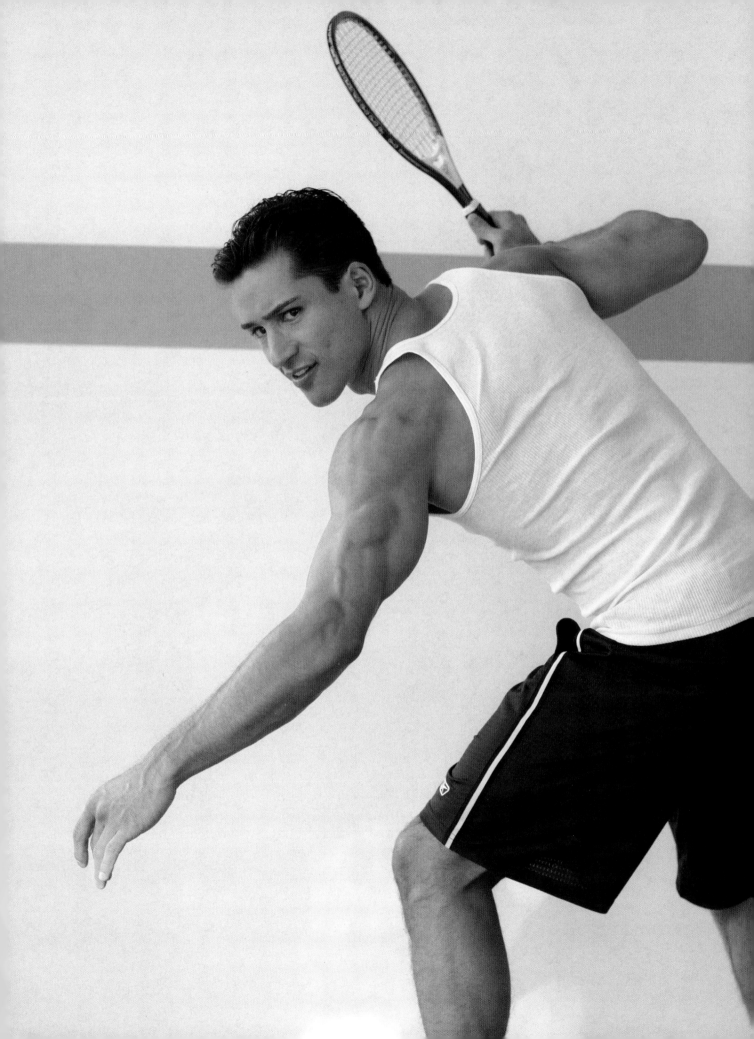

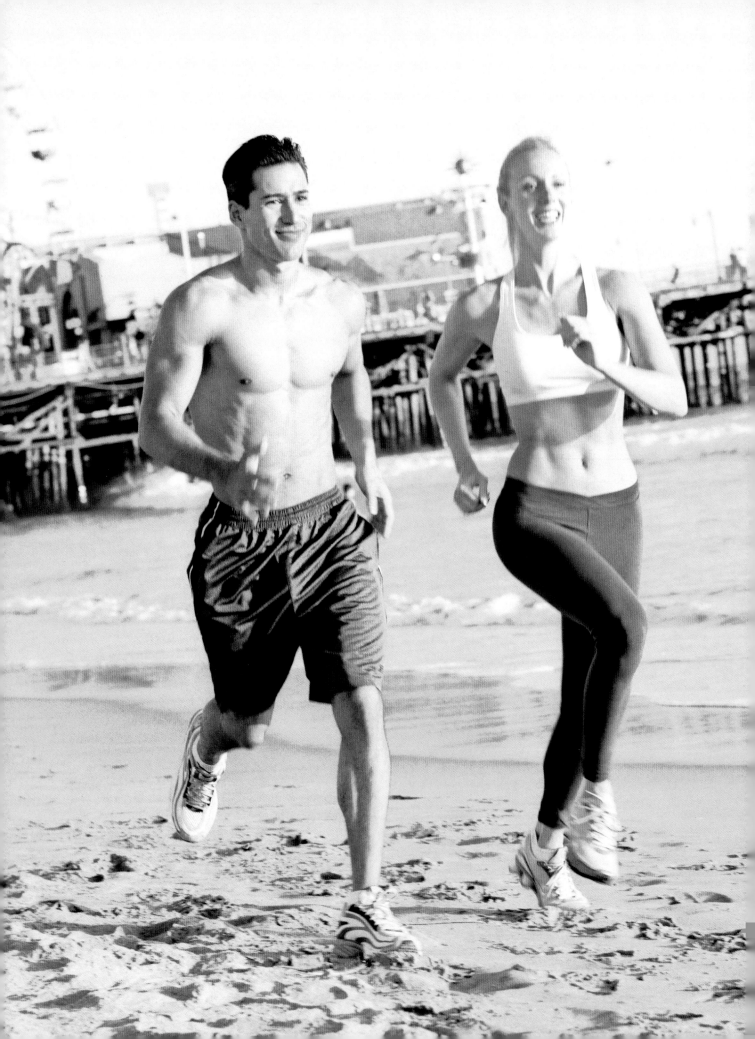

6 Meal Plans

My approach to eating is less about dieting and more about food scheduling. It's not Atkins, where carbohydrates are Public Enemy No. 1. It's not a low-fat diet, where you're never, ever allowed to eat, say, ribs. Heck, I love ribs. I don't do those blanket eliminations. That's why you won't feel like you're on a diet, in the conventional sense of that term. This will dramatically increase the odds of you sticking with it.

Yes, the Phase II meal plans include fewer calories, lower carb counts, and more protein than the Phase I plans. But you won't be starving yourself. On the contrary: You'll still be eating six or seven meals a day, keeping you feeling full despite the drops in calories and carbs. Breakfast options remain similar to the delicious choices in Phase I. Even when going low-carb, start your day with quality protein and healthy carbs, which are also strategically placed after your workouts. This energy will propel you through the day and help your body recover from tough-as-nails workouts, yet still allow your body to Pac-Man any rogue fat. The carbs do taper off as the day unfolds, which will only force your body to gobble up more body fat. The more you burn, the leaner you become.

You can still build muscle despite dropping calories by keeping your protein intake high. Although this isn't a high-protein diet, it is a diet that emphasizes protein. The reasons go beyond the fact that protein produces every hormone in your body, every enzyme, every disease-fighting antibody, and all the muscles that allow you to stand up and move around. Research has shown protein raises your metabolic rate higher than carbohydrate or fat does, and that it also slows the digestion of carbs to a crawl. That lowers insulin levels and decreases fat storage. It also raises levels of the hormones that blunt hunger.

Likewise, fat helps keep hunger in check, provides an additional energy source, and makes you feel good mentally. So fat remains at the Phase I level.

Before we go any further, I want to say a few words about cheat meals. If you fly 747s or perform laser-eye surgery, people have every right to expect—no, demand—perfection. In those endeavors, a batting average of 1.000 is mandatory. Make one mistake, and the end of your career is the least of your concerns. But eating? There, no one needs to be infallible. Nobody else eats perfectly, so why should you have to measure up against a standard that doesn't exist in the real world? People *think* it exists, but even those hard bodies you see at the gym and at the beach—the people who look like they've never tasted a slice of pizza in their entire life—cheat once in a while. Perhaps more often than you think. No, they don't make a video of themselves eating a jelly doughnut and then throw it up on YouTube for all the world to see. It's a clandestine indulgence. But it happens.

Their secret is twofold: a) they don't eat right all the time, but they eat right most of the time; and b) they almost certainly exercise regularly. It's like magic: When you're training regularly, all of sudden, your diet starts to forgive your mistakes. Taking a little side trip to Taco Bell? Hey, no problem. After all, tomorrow's leg day. And the yummy Cinnabon that would have headed straight to your love handles—all 813 calories and 32 grams of fat of it—gets torched on the treadmill instead. Icing on the cake, indeed.

The *occasional* cheat meal is one of the best ways to stick with a nutritional program long term. You don't have to be a dietary saint every day; a sin here or there won't undo what you've done previously. These cheat meals function as lights at the end of a tunnel, helping you make it through the week without surrendering to your cravings. After all, you know a reward is coming. Another reason to cheat has to do with your hormones. (And I'm not

HEY MARIO!

Name something I can do outside the gym to burn more calories!

Rely less on your car and escalators and more on your legs for daily transport. Work on the seventh floor of an office building? Walking up and down several times a day will burn calories. When you're trying to lose two pounds a week, burning off an additional 100 calories here or there from lifestyle choices makes a difference.

talking testosterone and estrogen here. What I'm about to say applies equally to men and women.) One of these hormones, lecithin, helps control metabolism, and it's very sensitive to carbohydrate intake. Think of lecithin as your body's fuel gauge, and carbohydrates as gasoline. When you go super-duper-low-carb, lecithin levels start decreasing, slowing down your metabolism. That's why when you do go low-carb, it's important to jack up the carbs one day out of every five or six. That kicks your lecithin levels back up, and jumpstart your metabolism.

So enjoy a cheat meal now and then. I sure do. Just don't go crazy on me, okay? At that one cheat meal, feel free to eat pretty much anything you want, within reason. You shouldn't eat an *entire* large pizza by yourself, but you can enjoy a few slices if that's what you're craving that night. Maybe it's my Catholic upbringing, but if I cheat too much, I feel guilty the next day. That's why I also

7 WAYS TO AVOID FOOD POISONING

1) Buy perishable foods last at the supermarket. Ask for ice if you have a long ride home. If you plan to make other stops after the grocery store, bring a cooler to keep perishable foods safe.

2) Wash your hands after arriving home and before preparing food. Wash them again after touching raw meats, fish, or eggs, to protect against germs, bacteria, or both being transferred among foods. There's no way to be 100 percent safe from food-borne infections, but washing your hands and cooking surfaces is the best insurance.

3) Clean your cutting board. Never use the same board for different foods without sanitizing it in between. Kill bacteria by running it through the dishwasher or rinsing it with a diluted chlorine solution (1 tablespoon of beach for 1 gallon of water). Try keeping one board for produce and another for raw meats, seafood, and poultry.

4) Avoid the danger zone! Keep cold foods under 40 degrees and hot foods above 140. Beware: In between lies trouble. To avoid it, use the fridge set lower than 40 degrees Fahrenheit. At 50 to 55 degrees, you have an incubator, not a refrigerator. On the flip side, reheat things thoroughly. Never leave foods out on the counter or outside, either. Bacteria will break out their party hats and go to town.

5) Don't work the blender like Rocky. No offense, Sly, but while eggs are a great source of high-quality protein, eating them raw or undercooked increases your risk of salmonella.

6) Thaw meat like a pro. Never defrost meat on the counter or in a pot of still water. Food-safety experts recommend using the refrigerator, the microwave, or cold running water. Unlike water sitting in a pot, running water will slow bacteria that could otherwise grow on the outer thawed portions, while the inside is still thawing.

7) Cook well. Here are the recommended internal temperatures (in degrees Fahrenheit): ground beef, 160; steak (medium rare), 145; chicken and turkey, 165; ground lamb, 160; lamb steaks, 145; pork, 160; leftovers of any kind, 165. If you're using a bone-in product—particularly like a whole bird—take the temperature in the thickest part of the thigh. That tends to be the coldest point.

don't go overboard with the cheat meals. To sculpt your best body, eat clean and healthfully 80 to 90 percent of the time. (What does "clean and healthfully" mean? Read the meal plans in this book and you'll know straight away.) Fall somewhere in that range, and your body will stay on track.

For many people, the damage from cheat days does more harm to their

10 HEALTHY ITEMS TO ADD TO YOUR SALAD

1) Avocado. This fruit—yes, technically it's a fruit—provides 25 different nutrients (including vitamins E and C), fiber, and hefty dose of healthy monounsaturated fats. Even better, it adds a unique buttery flavor to any salad. That way you don't have to pile on a high-calorie, nutrient-lacking creamy dressing.

2) Spinach. Rather than laying the rest of your salad on a bed of low-nutrient iceberg lettuce, use dark green spinach. It packs a hefty dose of iron, folate, and other nutrients with virtually no calories. Remember, the darker the color of a veggie or fruit, the better it is for you. That's never truer than with spinach.

3) Grapes. Whether red or black, these little nuggets are packed with health-boosting nutrients, particularly antioxidants called flavonoids. One of them, resveratrol, has been shown to lower the risk of heart disease. Grapes' crunchy texture and dry, sweet, tart, flavor make them a perfect salad topping.

4) Shiitake mushrooms. Yes, it's a fungus. So what? They contain nutrients that help boost the immune system, ward off cancer, and help you lose weight.

5) Wild blueberries. They're more diminutive than the blueberries normally seen on store shelves, but don't let that fool you. When it comes to disease-fighting antioxidants, they pack a real punch. Data from Tufts University suggests that anthocyanins, the antioxidants that make blueberries blue, boost your brain power.

6) Wild salmon. The omega 3 fats contained in salmon make you less prone to heart disease, Alzheimer's, joint pain, and a whole host of other maladies. Omega 3 fats help burn your body fat, too, while offering healthy amounts of iron, zinc, and protein.

7) Kidney beans. Like blueberries, these red beans contain enough antioxidants to gobble up nasty free radicals. What's more, 1/2 cup provides nearly half of the recommended daily dose of fiber, high amounts of iron and magnesium, and muscle-building protein for good measure.

8) Raw pecans. These are unusually high in antioxidants—for starters. They also supply ample amounts of monounsaturated fats, iron, selenium, and other vitamins and minerals. They even have a respectable amount of protein. Watch your portion size, though: A small handful packs on serious calories.

9) Red onions. They have a sweet taste and a strong smell—which is what makes them so healthful. Cutting them releases many of the nutrients, so chop finely. Red onions also supply chromium, which helps modulate blood sugar.

10) Broccoli. This vegetable provides well over 100 percent of the RDA of vitamin C. It also contains loads of fiber, vitamin K, vitamin A, and fiber. Better yet, a 2007 study published in the *Journal of the National Cancer Institute* concluded that high intake of vegetables such as broccoli may even reduce the risk of prostate cancer.

psyche than it does to their physique. They think, *Oh, my God—I've blown it, that's it*, so they binge for a week or two. Instead say, "Okay, that's done. Water under the bridge. Now I'm back on track." The bottom line is that the more cheat meals you allow yourself, the longer it will take you to reach your goal. This isn't rocket science. But we're all human, and if it takes a few more cheat days for you to not give up, go for it.

When you encounter the nutrition plan for Phase II, you'll notice that we've included some meals that look like cheat meals: chocolate squares with peanut butter, waffles topped with strawberries, even meals from Subway, KFC, and McDonald's (And as I've mentioned before these fast-food meals are all interchangeable with each other). You're probably thinking, *Can I really eat that stuff—during a phase when I'm supposed to be shedding fat and adding muscle?* Yes—you can even eat out when going lower carb. We provide several simple alternatives, as well as a few quick and easy frozen meals. These tasty options can be zapped in the microwave at home or in the office, requiring little effort on your part. Dieting doesn't get much easier than that.

Here's how your eating will shake out in Phase II. On those days when you're not working out, your body needs the following:

HEY MARIO!
I want lose 10 pounds for my high school reunion. How can I juggle my carb intake to maximize fat loss—stat?

Consume starchy carbs early in the day and water-rich carbs later. Your insulin sensitivity is greatest in the morning and falls off during the evening. So something like white rice will do more damage at dinner than it will at lunch. That's why you should eat those carbs that are absorbed more slowly by the body, like broccoli, later in the day.

- Anywhere from 9 to 11 calories per pound of body weight
- 0.5 grams of carbs per pound of body weight
- At least 1 gram of protein per pound of body weight
- 0.5 grams of fat per pound of body weight. Feel free to go a little higher.

9–11 calories × (your weight) = calories per day
.05 grams of carbs × (your weight) = carbohydrates per day
1 gram of protein × (your weight) = protein per day
0.5 grams of fat per pound (your weight) = fat per day

On workout days, your body needs the following:

- About 12 calories per pound of body weight
- A little more than 0.75 grams of carbs per pound of body weight
- A little more than 1 gram of protein per pound of body weight
- About 0.5 grams of fat per pound of body weight. Feel free to go a little higher.

This can be achieved simply by adding one snack to your diet from our "Workout Eats" section. Consume it as soon as possible after you work out.

12 calories × (your weight) = calories per day
>0.75 grams of carbs × (your weight) = carbohydrates per day
>1 gram of protein × (your weight) = protein per day
0.5 grams of fat per pound × (your weight) = fat per day

HEY MARIO!

I know what carbs I should avoid now: white bread, soda, sugary cereals, white rice, and so on. Name some healthy carb foods.

Sweet potatoes are my personal favorite, but the list is actually quite long: brown rice, oatmeal, and whole grains such as millet, quinoa, and wild rice all earn my seal of approval. And as a general rule, fruit provides good morning carbs, and vegetables provide good afternoon and evening carbs.

The following sample meal plans represent what I typically eat. But if you weigh less than 175 pounds, you'll want to reduce your intake. One way is to cut out one of the three daily snacks. For example, if you don't feel hungry between breakfast and lunch, skip the late-morning snack. Alternatively, reduce your overall calorie intake by using smaller serving sizes for some meals. To cut back on protein, for example, eat two eggs instead of four at breakfast. You can also eat less deli meat, $\frac{1}{2}$ cup of cottage cheese instead of 1 cup, or a smaller portion of protein (chicken, turkey, seafood, or steak) at dinner. To cut back on your carbohydrate intake, eat half a bagel or English muffin instead of a whole one, and $\frac{1}{2}$ cup of cereal instead of 1 cup.

Workout Eats

You should adopt the habit of refueling your energy stores and feeding your muscles after exercising them. So on training days, consume one of these snacks as soon as possible but within an hour after your workout.

Food	Calories	Protein (g)	Carbs (g)	Fat (g)
Power Bar Protein Plus	270	22	30	9
Clif Builder	270	20	30	8
16 oz. Jamba Juice Protein Berry Workout w/ soy protein	280	14	56	1
16 oz low-fat chocolate milk	316	16	52	4
8 oz plain non-fat yogurt + 1 cup blueberries	210	14	38	0

Sample Daily Meal Plans: Phase II
Monday

Breakfast

2 whole eggs

2 egg whites

Fry or scramble using non-fat cooking spray.

3 slices Jennie-O extra lean turkey bacon

1 packet Lower Sugar Quaker Instant Oatmeal (flavored: maple and brown sugar or apples and cinnamon)

Late-morning snack

1 cup cottage cheese

¼ cup sliced pineapple

Mix pineapple into cottage cheese.

Lunch

Lean Cuisine Roasted Garlic Chicken

Mid-afternoon snack

4 ounces plain low-fat yogurt

1 tablespoon peanut butter

Mix peanut butter into yogurt.

Dinner

9 ounces salmon (broiled or grilled)

½ cup mixed vegetables (canned or frozen), prepared

8 bittersweet (60% cacao) chocolate chips

1 tablespoon peanut butter

Mix chocolate chips into peanut butter.

Late-night snack

1 cup cottage cheese

2 tablespoons salsa

Top cottage cheese with salsa.

Totals: 1,906 calories, 83 grams of carbohydrates, 185 grams of protein, 89 grams of fat.

* If you work out today, choose one snack from "Workout Eats," and consume within one hour of working out. Be sure to consider these nutritional values when planning your nutrition totals for the day.

Tuesday

Breakfast

Breakfast burrito

2 whole eggs

2 egg whites

1 slice low-fat American cheese

2 slices low-fat deli ham

10-inch whole-wheat tortilla

Heat tortilla in warm pan. Fry ham in pan, and place on tortilla; whisk eggs and scramble in pan using non-stick cooking spray; add cheese and place on tortilla; roll into breakfast burrito.

Late-morning snack

1 ounce fat-free cheese (Swiss, cheddar, Monterey jack, etc.)

2 slice (2 ounces) turkey deli meat

Slice cheese into two thin pieces and place in middle of turkey. Roll up turkey and eat.

1 ounce mixed nuts

Lunch

McDonald's Tendergrill Chicken Salad (use ½ packet light Italian dressing)

Mid-afternoon snack

½ can tuna

½ cup low-fat cottage cheese

Mix tuna and cottage cheese.

Dinner

Taco salad

4 ounces lean ground beef (95% lean; lean ground turkey is an acceptable substitute)

1 teaspoon taco seasoning

¼ cup shredded fat-free cheddar cheese

1 tablespoon fat-free sour cream

4 tablespoons salsa

1 cup shredded iceberg lettuce

½ medium tomato, diced

Brown meat; add taco seasoning; place meat over lettuce bed; add tomato, cheese, salsa and sour cream.

½ cup blueberries

2 tablespoons fat-free Reddi Wip

Top blueberries with Reddi Wip.

Late-night snack

2 ounces beef jerky

Totals: 1,639 calories, 86 grams of carbohydrates, 185 grams of protein, 59 grams of fat.

* If you work out today, choose one snack from "Workout Eats," and consume within one hour of working out. Be sure to consider these nutritional values when planning your nutrition totals for the day.

Wednesday

Breakfast

Western Bagel Healthy Grain Bagel (Perfect 10 Bagel)

1 tablespoon peanut butter

Spread peanut butter on bagel.

Late-morning snack

8 ounces reduced-fat Greek yogurt (2%)

½ medium cucumber, diced

Dill (optional)

Add cucumber slices to yogurt, and add dill, if desired.

Lunch

Turkey & avocado rolls

4 slices turkey deli meat

4 slices low-fat American cheese

½ avocado

1 tablespoon light mayonnaise

Layer 1 slice of cheese on 1 slice of turkey for four separate breadless sandwiches. Spread mayo on cheese. Slice avocado into 4 strips and put 1 slice of avocado in middle of each slice of cheese. Roll meat and cheese around avocado.

Mid-afternoon snack

4 ounces shrimp

1 tablespoon seafood cocktail sauce

Dip shrimp in cocktail sauce.

Dinner

8 ounces chicken breast (baked or grilled)

1 cup Progresso Healthy Classics Beef Vegetable soup

1 Edy's/Dreyer's Frozen Fruit Bar (strawberry, tangerine, or raspberry)

Late-night snack

2 ounces fat-free cheese (Swiss, cheddar, or Monterey jack)

2 or 3 large celery stalks

1 tablespoon peanut butter

Spoon peanut butter into groove of celery.

Totals: 1,688 calories, 85 grams of carbohydrates, 190 grams of protein, 69 grams of fat.

* If you work out today, choose one snack from "Workout Eats," and consume within one hour of working out. Be sure to consider these nutritional values when planning your nutrition totals for the day.

Thursday

Breakfast

Spinach & cheese omelet

2 whole eggs

2 egg whites

2 tablespoons light cream cheese

1/2 cup chopped raw spinach

1 teaspoon olive oil

Whisk the eggs and cook in a pan with olive oil or non-fat cooking spray. Flip eggs. Mix cream cheese and spinach in a bowl. Spread cream cheese mixture onto cooked side of egg. Wait 30 seconds to ensure the other side of the egg is fully cooked. Fold in half. Wait 1 minute to melt cream cheese mixture.

1 whole-wheat English muffin

1 tablespoon peanut butter

Late-morning snack

2 hard-boiled eggs

2 to 3 large celery stalks

1 tablespoon peanut butter

Spoon peanut butter into groove of celery.

Lunch

1/2 can tuna

1 tablespoon light mayonnaise

3 whole-wheat crackers

Pickle relish and chopped vegetables (optional)

Mix tuna with mayo. If desired, add pickle relish and vegetables. Eat with crackers.

Mid-afternoon snack

8 ounces reduced-fat Greek yogurt (2%)

1/8 cup shelled sunflower seeds

Mix sunflower seeds into yogurt.

Dinner

6 ounces top sirloin steak (grilled or broiled)

1 cup cooked cauliflower

2 cups mixed green salad

1 tablespoon olive oil-and-vinegar salad dressing

2 squares (2 ounces) dark chocolate (60 to 70% cacao)

1 teaspoon peanut butter

Spread peanut butter on chocolate.

Late-night snack

2 ounces beef jerky

Totals: 1,957 calories, 90 grams of carbohydrates, 164 grams of protein, 104 grams of fat.

＊ If you work out today, choose one snack from "Workout Eats," and consume within one hour of working out. Be sure to consider these nutritional values when planning your nutrition totals for the day.

Friday

Breakfast

1 cup Kashi GoLean Cereal
4 ounces skim milk
Eat cereal with milk.

2 hard-boiled eggs

Late-morning snack

½ cup boiled soybeans (edamame)
1 stick light mozzarella string cheese (1 ounce)

Lunch

Subway Oven Roasted Chicken Salad (double meat with 1 teaspoon red wine vinaigrette dressing)

Mid-afternoon snack

6 ounces shrimp
1 teaspoon seafood cocktail sauce

Dinner

Chili con carne

6 ounces lean ground beef (95% lean; lean ground turkey is an acceptable substitute)
¼ can diced tomatoes
¼ medium onion
½ teaspoon ground cumin powder
1 teaspoon chili powder
Brown beef in pan. Add tomatoes, onion, ground cumin powder, and chili powder. Add salt and pepper to taste.

2 squares (2 ounces) dark chocolate (60 to 70% cacao)
1 teaspoon peanut butter
Spread peanut butter on chocolate.

Late-night snack

2 sticks light mozzarella string cheese (2 ounces)

2 or 3 large celery stalks
1 tablespoon peanut butter
Spoon peanut butter into groove of celery

Totals: 1,640 calories, 96 grams of carbohydrates, 178 grams of protein, 64 grams of fat.

* If you work out today, choose one snack from "Workout Eats," and consume within one hour of working out. Be sure to consider these nutritional values when planning your nutrition totals for the day.

Saturday

Breakfast

Cheese omelet

2 whole eggs and 2 egg whites

¼ cup fat-free cheddar cheese

Scramble eggs. Pour in pan over medium heat with fat-free cooking spray. Flip egg. Add cheese. Fold over to make omelet.

1 whole-grain waffle

½ cup sliced strawberries

1 tablespoon fat-free sour cream

1 teaspoon brown sugar

Mix sugar into sour cream. Add strawberries to waffle. Top with sour cream.

Late-morning snack

½ cup plain low-fat yogurt

1 tablespoon peanut butter

Mix peanut butter into yogurt.

Lunch

Dijon tuna salad

2 tablespoons white wine vinegar

1 teaspoon Dijon mustard

1 tablespoon olive oil

½ can tuna

2 cups mixed green salad

In a microwave-safe bowl, place vinegar and mustard and mix. Add olive oil and tuna and mix. Microwave for 1 minute until warm. Pour over salad.

Mid-afternoon snack

2 slices low-fat American cheese

4 slices low-fat deli ham

Lay 1 slice of cheese between two slices of ham. Roll up.

1 ounce walnuts (14 halves)

1 teaspoon peanut butter

Dinner

Chicken divan

8 ounces chicken breast

1 cup chopped broccoli

½ can 98% fat-free cream of mushroom soup

Brown chicken in pan with non-fat cooking spray. Add broccoli, cook for 5 to 10 minutes. Add soup and cook 5 to 10 minutes. Top with cheese.

½ cup sliced strawberries

2 tablespoons fat-free Reddi Wip

Top strawberries with Reddi Wip.

Late-night snack

1 cup cottage cheese

2 tablespoons salsa

Top cottage cheese with salsa.

Totals: 1,900 calories, 94 grams of carbohydrates, 192 grams of protein, 86 grams of fat.

* If you work out today, choose one snack from "Workout Eats," and consume within one hour of working out. Be sure to consider these nutritional values when planning your nutrition totals for the day.

Sunday

Breakfast

Western Bagel Healthy Grain Bagel (Perfect 10 Bagel)

1 tablespoon peanut butter

Late-morning snack

2 hard-boiled eggs

$\frac{1}{2}$ large grapefruit

Lunch

1 KFC grilled chicken breast

1 side order green beans

House side salad with $\frac{1}{2}$ packet Hidden Valley Ranch dressing

Mid-afternoon snack

$\frac{1}{2}$ can tuna

$\frac{1}{2}$ cup low-fat cottage cheese

Mix tuna into cottage cheese.

Dinner

Shrimp stir-fry

1 cup frozen stir-fry vegetables

6 ounces shrimp

1 tablespoon soy sauce

Spray non-fat cooking spray in frying pan. Heat to medium high and add vegetables. Cook, stirring occasionally until vegetables have begun to thaw (about 5 minutes). Add shrimp and soy sauce, continue cooking until shrimp is pink and tender.

2 cups mixed green salad

1 tablespoon olive oil-and-vinegar salad dressing

$\frac{1}{2}$ cup blueberries

2 tablespoons fat-free Reddi Wip

Top blueberries with Reddi Wip.

Late-night snack

1 stick light mozzarella string cheese (1 ounce)

2 ounces beef jerky

Totals: 1,592 calories, 90 grams of carbohydrates, 168 grams of protein, 62 grams of fat.

* If you work out today, choose one snack from "Workout Eats," and consume within one hour of working out. Be sure to consider these nutritional values when planning your nutrition totals for the day.

QUICK & TASTY MEALS

Breakfast

Oatmeal with Stewed Fruit

1 cup dried apricots
1 cup dried pears
1 cup dried prunes
1 tablespoon brown sugar
1 teaspoon ground cinnamon
3 cups water

Combine all ingredients in a saucepan. Bring to a boil, cover and simmer for 20 minutes until fruit is plumped and liquid is slightly thickened.

Makes 4 1-cup servings.

Add 1 cup stewed fruit, 1½ cups cooked oatmeal; tea with ¼ cup skim milk.

Total: 482 calories; 13 grams protein, 104 grams carbohydrates, 4 grams fat (11% protein, 82% carbohydrates, 7% fat)

Lunch & Dinner
1,000 calories

Salmon with Curry Sauce

Vegetable cooking spray
1 pound salmon fillets, rinsed and patted dry
1 tablespoon plus 1 teaspoon canola oil
1 tablespoon chopped chives
1 tablespoon curry powder
1 teaspoon dry mustard
¼ cup white wine
2 tablespoons lemon juice
1 tablespoon dried currants
1 teaspoon cornstarch, dissolved in ¾ cup evaporated skimmed milk

Spray a broiler pan with vegetable cooking spray. Brush fillets with 1 teaspoon of canola oil and broil about 10 minutes per inch of fish. In a small skillet, heat 1 tablespoon oil. Add chives, curry powder, and mustard, and blend thoroughly. Remove from heat; stirring constantly, add wine and lemon juice. Return to heat and add currants. Stir cornstarch mixture into curry mixture and blend. Remove broiled fish and top with curry sauce.

Makes 2 servings.

Add 2 cups tossed salad; 2 tablespoons Light Ranch dressing; 1 cup boiled cauliflower; 1 cup cooked brown rice; 1 fat-free pudding cup with 4 tablespoons Cool Whip Lite; water or Crystal Light.

Total: 1,000 calories; 67 grams protein, 103 grams carbohydrates, 35 grams fat (27% protein, 41% carbohydrates, 32% fat)

Lunch & Dinner
500 calories

Blackened Tuna Steaks

1 tablespoon onion powder
1 tablespoon fried whole basil
2 teaspoons dried whole thyme
$\frac{1}{2}$ teaspoon ground white pepper
$\frac{1}{8}$ to $\frac{1}{4}$ teaspoon ground red pepper
$\frac{1}{2}$ teaspoon black pepper
6 (4 ounce) tuna steaks
Vegetable cooking spray
$1\frac{1}{2}$ tablespoons margarine, melted

Combine onion powder, basil, thyme, white pepper, red pepper and black pepper in a small bowl and stir well. Rub steaks with pepper mixture. Coat grill rack with cooking spray and place on grill over medium-hot coals. Place tuna on rack; drizzle with margarine and cook 4 to 5 minutes on each side or until tuna flakes easily when tested with a fork.

Makes 6 servings.

Add 1 cup chicken noodle soup; $\frac{1}{2}$ cup cooked brown rice; 1 cup cooked mixed frozen vegetables; 1 cup sugar-free Jell-O; water or Crystal Light.

Total: 498 calories; 39 grams protein, 57 grams carbohydrates, 12 grams fat (32% protein, 46% carbohydrates, 22% fat)

Snacks

Cottage Cheese and Fruit

$\frac{1}{2}$ cup no-sugar-added canned fruit
$\frac{1}{2}$ cup cottage cheese (1% fat)

119 calories; 14 grams protein, 13 grams carbohydrates, 1 gram fat (48% protein, 43% carbohydrates, 9% fat)

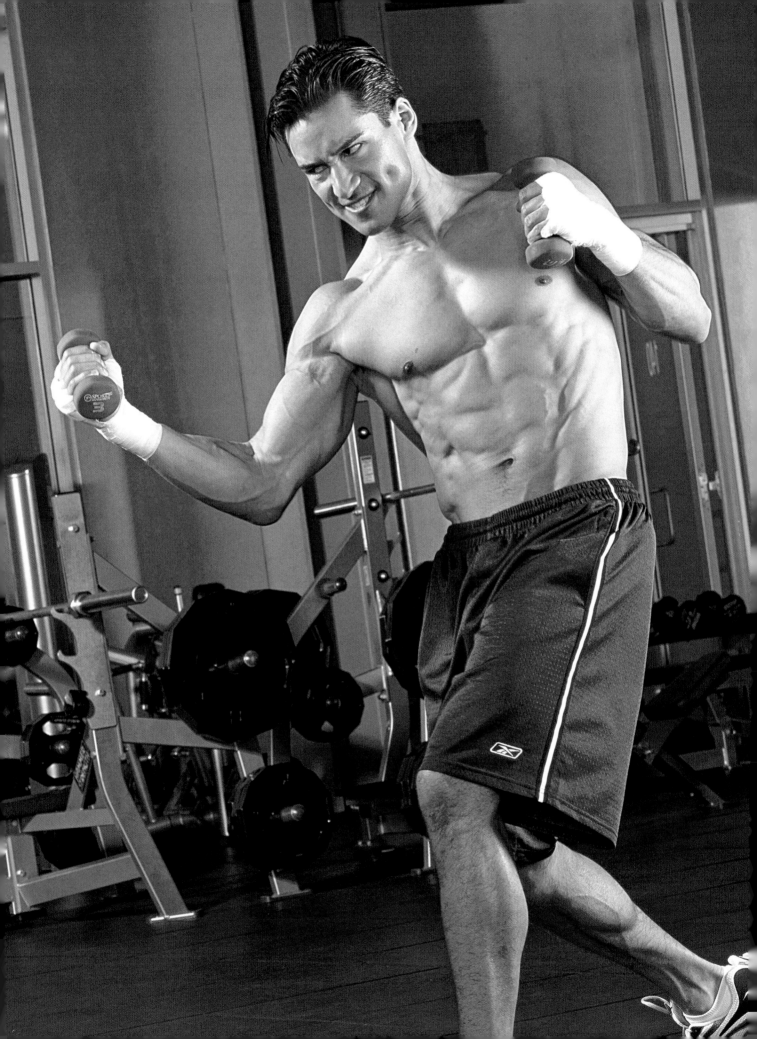

7 The Shape of Your Life

Aim high in the gym, and you can aim higher in life. Opportunity knocks; one door opens the next; there's more room to grow than you can possibly imagine. You'll be able to do things once you're in shape that you don't even realize yet.

Don't let naysayers tell you otherwise. In reality, there's nothing you *can't* do once you set your mind to it and take action.

I'm living proof of that.

Believe me, there was no silver spoon in my mouth when I was born on October 10, 1973. I'm a first-generation American from Chula Vista, California, north of San Diego. I come from a very hard-working, blue-collar family. There were no performers in my family. My father, Mario, Sr., worked for the city; my mother, Elvira, for the phone company. The logical trajectory for me wasn't to enter the entertainment field.

Growing up, I was a very hyper kid. I was always running around and getting banged up: a broken nose, scars everywhere—the whole nine yards. The neighborhood where we lived was full of roughnecks on the lookout for trouble. I was a standup kid who stood on his own two feet, but my mom put two and two together and realized that she needed to channel my energy constructively, in order to keep me off the streets and out of trouble. So she guided me into wrestling, karate practice, and parts in little school plays. Acting came easily to me for several reasons. First, I was a smart kid and could read really well for my age. (In fact, I had been reading since the age of 3.) What's more, I was very outgoing and not at all shy around adults. Precocious is the word, I think.

I was competing in a talent competition as a 10-year-old when my mom overheard a local talent agent talking to another lady about her kid. A light bulb clicked in my mom's head: *Hey, my kid can do that!* She asked me what I thought about the idea. I was like, "Yeah, sounds fun. Why not?" I certainly wasn't shy, and it was something else to do. So, from that moment on, she campaigned for me to join their agency. To appreciate what that meant, you'd have to meet my mom, who's a very determined lady. Eventually, the woman met me, liked me, and signed me up. I was in show biz.

HEY, MARIO!
Does a lower-intensity activity such as walking really do a better job of burning fat than a higher-intensity activity such as sprinting?
This is sort of a trick question. True, a higher percentage of the calories burned for fuel come from fat while walking. But the absolute number of fat calories burned is lower because you torch so many more *total* calories by sprinting. Walking on a treadmill for an hour, maybe you burn 300 calories, with 200 from fat. Work harder, and those numbers rise to, say, 600 and 250, respectively. I'll take the latter.

Next thing you know, I began doing print work and commercials. It became like having an after-school activity every day. Some kids go to little league practice; some kids go to clarinet practice; I went to auditions. I just kind of did what my mom told me. If I had an interview or casting to attend, cool; if I didn't, that was cool, too. I'd be off doing something else, like wrestling. My parents never pressured me, never once tried to live vicariously through my experiences. Acting and modeling were just two more activities among many that I pursued.

Looking back, I took things some people might have predicted to become liabilities—hyperactivity and a short attention span—and turned them into assets. I've taken that same approach repeatedly ever since. If I've had one secret to success in my life to date, that's it. It's something you can do in the gym, too, by following these workouts: take your body from liability to asset.

After doing a series of small, local gigs in and around San Diego, I began traveling north to Los Angeles for auditions. Hollywood, here I come. One thing led to another, and soon I was starring on *Kids Incorporated*, a variety show where many future stars, including Fergie and Martika, found their start. (It was sort of a modern-day version of *The Mickey Mouse Club*.) I did that show for three and a half years, all the while continuing to do a bunch of commercials and print work. I would also guest on shows such as *The Golden Girls*.

Talk about a juggling act—all the while, I was still attending junior high school near San Diego, and then starting my freshman year at Chula Vista High School. I played on the football team for one season, but the sporadic nature of my schedule made it tough for me to contribute. It's not fair to your teammates to never know if you'll be there. So I turned my attention to high school wrestling instead. Being an individual sport, that was much easier for me to pursue.

Wrestling competitively was the first time that I really became conscious of body weight. They often talk about how the requirements of gymnastics makes young girls acutely aware of their size—often too aware, which can lead to eating disorders. Well, wrestling makes guys obsess over the scales, if only because they wrestle in weight classes, and you need to make weight. Try having to shed three pounds overnight so that you can compete the next day in your weight class. That's pressure.

The intersection of wrestling, body weight, and food probably took on even greater significance for me because I come from a Hispanic family. Mothers like mine want their sons to be really thick; that's considered the ideal, not a problem needing a remedy.

Mexican cuisine might be the best-tasting food in the world, but it's not necessarily the healthiest, at least not the way it's traditionally made. You can cook it in a healthy way, but my mom and grandmother were not ones to abide by that. They would cook in lard and use other techniques that were old-school. But, man, it tasted good, I'll tell you that.

There would be guys walking around all huge at 175 pounds who would wrestle in meets at 160, but my family didn't like me cutting weight even four pounds. Back then, you'd hear horror stories about guys cutting weight, a practice that isn't healthy for a young man. So in retrospect, I'm grateful to my parents for their disapproval. Maybe I wrestled bigger guys, but at least I was healthy, eating what I wanted, and training hard.

If I was an unlikely wrestler, I was a less likely actor. It would have been very easy for me assume that nothing significant would come of my television work. Other than Desi Arnaz on *I Love Lucy*, I didn't see many people on television that looked like me. No one else seemed to have my skin color. I had to look elsewhere for my role models, to people within my community, like my wrestling coach and drama coach and parents, all of whom I admire and respect to this day. They shared one common denominator: They were all really hardworking people.

But my big break came when I landed the role of A.C. Slater on the Saturday morning sitcom *Saved by the Bell*. I was a sophomore at Chula Vista High when I landed that gig. Because everybody was a minor, we filmed during the summer. Bizarre, huh? Here you are acting as a high school student, but then you actually go back and become a real high school student year-round.

Despite being on a hit TV show, I was treated no differently back home by the kids I had grown up with in my neighborhood. I didn't go back and talk about anything. If you tried to be a showoff in my neighborhood, guys would put you in check real quick. So I laid low and minded my own business. Sure, if they asked about it, I would say something, but most of the time I would kind of blow it off and shift the conversation to other stuff. Also, I had carved out a reputation as a formidable wrestler, a guy who could handle himself in a scrape if need be. I think that gave me credibility that otherwise would have been lacking. It made me reputable.

My family helped keep me grounded as well. I'm very blessed to have parents that have been happily married for more than 35 years. When I was growing up, we were a very close-knit family. They just looked at acting as another activity that I did. I still had chores to do at home, still helped my dad out around the yard—you name it. They treated my sister and me exactly the same. I looked at the show as just a temporary job, because that's all any of them are in the end. No job is forever in TV. Everything from *Gunsmoke* to *Friends* comes to end eventually.

Fortunately for me, *Saved by the Bell* turned out to be a five-year temp job. That's how long the original run lasted, although it repeats in syndication seemingly every day. I was there from beginning to end. To this day, people still walk up and say, "Hey, you're A.C. Slater!" And that's cool. I'll take that as a compliment. If nothing else, I guess it means I haven't aged too poorly if they still recognize me, right? That show forms part of TV history now. *Saved by the Bell* has become *The Brady Bunch* of its generation. So I'm grateful to have had that opportunity and happy to have been a part of it.

In my 20s, it gradually dawned on me that I wanted to pursue this line of work for the rest of my life. It beat getting a real job, you know? (My dad still asks me when I'll get one of those.) But I also realized that it's probably the toughest line of work to last in. The odds against you making it are long, the competition fierce, the obstacles many. I didn't want to sit around by the phone, waiting for it to ring. (I'm too hyper anyway. I *needed* to be busy.) So I hustled. I wanted to host, I wanted to act, I wanted to do radio, I wanted to learn about production behind the scenes—all of the above. I tried to do everything. Fortunately, I haven't yet experienced a career lull, and I think it's because I've always been working in at least some facet of the business. If you just sit around and wait for your agent to call you, you're going to wind up going hungry a lot. That's probably the best piece of advice I can offer you aspiring entertainers out there. Make it happen.

I've often been asked to name my favorite part of the business, and I can honestly say that I like it all. I like working, staying busy. Whether it's subbing for Larry King or Regis or having a barbecue at my house, hosting comes naturally for me. I love people.

As I fashioned my career in show business, I found others whose own path in life inspired me, and who made me want to emulate some measure of their success. These modern-day role models have tended to be actors and hosts who also believe in giving back to the community. Oprah Winfrey started out as an actress, and a good one, and look where she is. Ellen DeGeneres and Kelly Ripa also balance hosting gigs with acting careers. Interestingly, there aren't too many guys, other than maybe Steve Harvey or someone like that, who do everything that I do: radio, TV, hosting, and acting.

And, again, they really go out and get after it. There's just no substitute for hard work, and that applies equally to your career and your fitness. I'm not saying you have to kill yourself in the process, but you must be willing to make the commitment to work hard in order to achieve anything of true significance in life. There are no shortcuts.

Like some of my role models, I too look for ways to give back. I just finished a big campaign for PepsiCo that I'm really proud of, for example. It was called The Smart Spot Campaign, and it focused on mothers and kids in the inner city, where obesity has become such an epidemic, especially among the Latino and African American communities. We're trying to help them shape up by offering nutrition tips and fun exercise programs that they can do at home. We went to

HEY, MARIO!
What's the best investment I can make in building my body?
Buying this book was a great start. Purchasing a gym membership is another. In fact, I'm not sure any investment beats 30 bucks a month or whatever for that privilege. Beyond that, I would say that I'm surprised tens of millions of people hire personal trainers and nearly no one hires a nutritionist, when nutrition is 80 percent of the battle. That's never made much sense to me.

practically every major city in America. I'm a former inner city kid myself, so I know from firsthand experience that in that environment, oftentimes you're just not privy to that type of information. As a society, we need to show these kids how to live a healthier lifestyle. We need to help them make good choices, beginning with what kind of food they put in their mouth.

One reason I'm sympathetic to people who are struggling to make their way in life is that I still feel like I could lose all of this at any moment. I *like* feeling that way, as strange as that might sound. It prevents complacency and keeps me from taking anything for granted. I've always had a hustling mentality and still have what you might call "guarded optimism." Stuff can go away at the snap of your fingers. That's why I'm a big saver, and that's why I try to work just as hard, if not harder, than I ever have before. I try to help out my family as much as I can, and I'm building for a family of my own one day as well. I'm

CHECKLIST FOR TOMORROW

I'm a compulsive note maker. I'm continuously jotting down short-term and long-term goals, to do lists, notes to self—you name it. I have a lot going in my life at any given moment, and if I didn't write stuff down, I'd forget half of what I need to do each day. By recording this information as it pops into my head—and that's key, because it will leave soon enough—I know it's there to be done, yet I can focus on the task at hand and stay in the moment.

The most important time to write stuff down is right before you go to sleep. I take ten minutes each night to outline my goals for the coming day. That way, when the alarm rings, I have a game plan outlining everything I need to do that day, just like one of those NFL coaches holding a plastic sheet listing all their plays. They've planned in advance. They don't just go out there and start throwing the ball around.

Here are some key elements to include in your checklist:

1) What key appointments do you have? Arrange them in your day so that you can meet them as expeditiously as possible.

2) What key errands do you need to run/accomplish? Schedule those so you're not wasting time, doubling back, etc.

3) What do you need to eat, and when? You have your meal plans in hand, so make sure you plan to execute them.

4) When do you plan to work out? Again, you have that in black and white now, but make sure you have time to complete your workout.

5) What else needs doing? Haven't called your mom in two weeks? Then schedule it!

just really appreciative of what's happening, and hoping it will all continue.

That notion that everything could end in a heartbeat is also why I'm so focused on planning for the future and career longevity. Which brings me to two other role models who've had a major positive impact on my life, and who I really look up to: Dick Clark and Merv Griffin. I worked with Dick on the talk show *The Other Half* several years ago, and I absorbed so much wisdom just from being around him. We're still good friends. He wrote me a very nice note just the other day, after seeing me host a TV show. Merv is another guy with whom I struck up a friendship. We were actually going to do a project together before his unfortunate passing.

Dick and Merv not only made names for themselves as hosts and in other entertainment venues, but they also pursued a wide range of successful business ventures. Dick owns a lot of real estate ventures and businesses all over the world, and so did Merv. Those are two guys who became successful on television but then really capitalized on it through their business savvy.

Your path will undoubtedly be different from mine. How could it not be? But the lessons I've learned and the obstacles I've overcome apply equally to anyone's life. First, don't think your circumstances dictate the trajectory of your life. I had loving, supportive parents, but nothing in my upbringing suggested that I would become what I am today. And nothing about being a child actor guaranteed that I'd still be going to strong today. (If you don't believe that—well, the headlines have spoken for themselves over the years). What I've done is dream big, yes, but I've also taken the necessary steps to realize those dreams. It's not enough to want something. You need to execute.

That's a lesson that working out reinforces for me every day. You want to look diesel? Great. It's awesome that you have that goal. But you have to do X, Y, and Z nearly every day to make it happen. Do it, and it will happen.

Second—and I alluded to this earlier—turn your liabilities into assets. For me, it was taking hyperactivity and making it work for me, not against me. (Even in the gym, I've built my training style around my short attention span.) If you don't look like a movie star, for example, find other ways to stand out. Cultivate your sense of humor. Build an interesting career. Become someone who others respect. It's the people who wallow in what they perceive to be their shortcomings who never achieve anything worthwhile. And half the time their limitations are all in their head anyway.

Third, stay grounded. This is another area where working out helps. No matter how much success you enjoy, the weights are still going to try and kick your butt every workout. After all, they have gravity on their side. Beyond that, don't forget where you came from, or lose sight of what's really important in life. Hint: It's not material things. Don't be one of those people who knows the price of everything and the value of nothing.

Last but not least, listen to those with more experience and wisdom than you have, whether it's a schoolteacher or a personal trainer at the gym. That's why I count Larry King and Dick Clark among my friends—I value what they have to say because their life experiences extend beyond my own at this point. We're becoming more and more disconnected from our past and it's a huge mistake. Those who don't learn the mistakes of the past are doomed to repeat them, as someone once said.

Which is why it's time to the junk the bogus workout programs you've followed in the past, and commit to one that actually works: mine!

Phase 3
Weeks 5 and 6

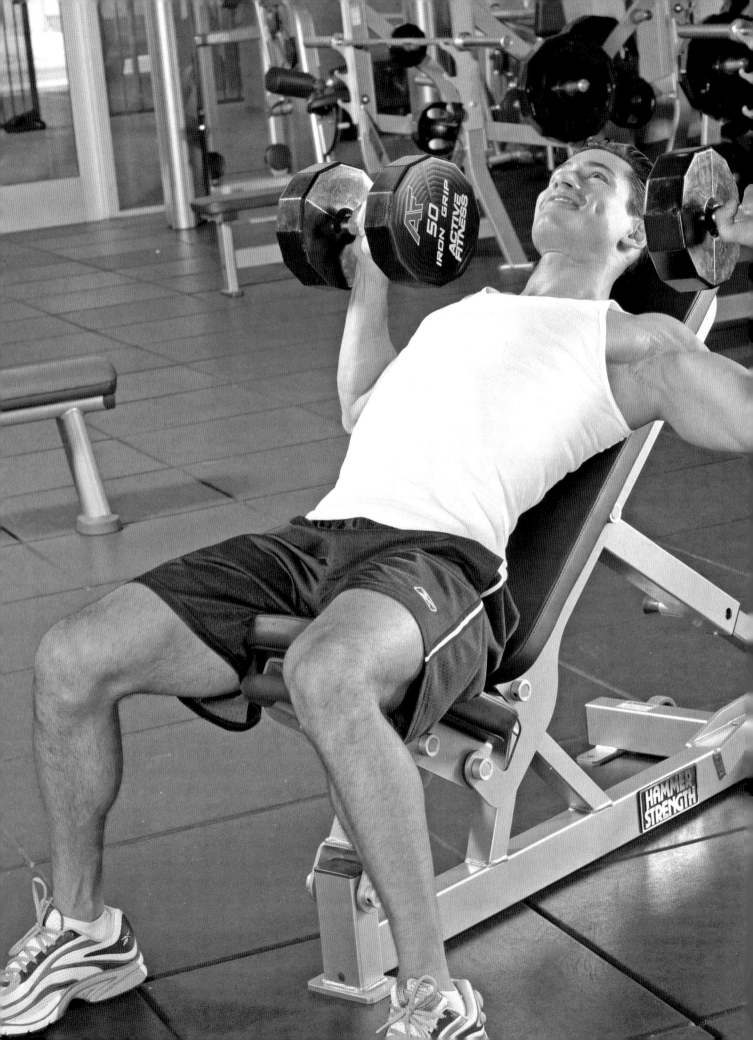

8 Max It Out!

In Phase III, you'll be performing not two weights-and-cardio workouts each week, but three. That's the primary difference between this phase and those preceding it. By now, you've developed a higher work capacity, so we're going to take advantage of that improvement by introducing a greater variety of exercises. The rep schemes also become a little more varied during this phase. One workout you'll be doing higher-volume work, meaning 12 to 15 reps per set. Then, *boom*, you'll be doing some 8-to-10s with longer rest periods, more of a classic muscle-building approach. And in the third workout of the week, get ready for some pure power movements. For example, that session begins with front squats followed by bench jumps. Later in the same workout, you'll be throwing around a medicine ball.

These moves might seem a little unconventional to you, but they're designed to develop strength and power. They work equally well for men and women, who are dealing in the realm of power every time they take a kickboxing class. Strength remains a caricature for many people, who associate it with hammers being swung at carnivals, or guys piling out into the backyard to see who can bench Dad's Monte Carlo. I doubt that many of you want to compete in strongman contests—more power to those of you who do—but everyone should attempt to become stronger. Among many other benefits, improved strength permits you to lift heavier weights, allowing for the building of more muscle. That increased muscle tone won't just turn guys' heads, ladies—it'll help you burn fat all day, even while you sleep! As I've explained before, more muscle translates into less fat.

During Phase III, you'll also improve your power, which refers to the application of strength at high velocities. When you throw a left hook during my boxing workout, that's power. When you dismount from a balance beam, that's power. You're taking the strength developed by working out and setting it in motion.

The more force you can move at high speeds, the more powerful you are. Whether you're talking about an ultimate fighter slamming an opponent to the canvas, a baseball player hitting a tape-measure home run, or a woman driving a backhand past her opponent, power is essential for success in nearly every sport. Except for maybe badminton. But I don't play that game.

Even workout buffs shy away from bench jumps, medicine ball tosses, and the like because they don't associate them with getting pumped, the way you would when doing 15 biceps curls in succession. That's a misconception. These moves work fast-twitch muscle fibers. We're not talking about a nervous tic here; on the contrary, fast-twitchers are the primary source of human power, but only if you know how to call them to arms in unison. At the Australian Institute of Sport, where many of the top Australian Olympians train, researchers found that when they added plyometrics to the workout routines of world-class distance runners, they were able to run five percent farther using the same amount of energy—after only nine weeks!

Fast-twitch muscle fibers are the first to go as you age, too. "We've seen biological evidence of muscle deterioration starting in a person's early thirties," says Mark Tarnopolsky, MD, PhD, a professor of medicine at McMaster University in Canada. The explosive-type moves we've added to the program will help stave off the slow decline toward weakness and osteoporosis.

Yet we don't want to lose those other qualities—muscle growth, muscular endurance, and so on—that you worked so hard and so diligently to develop in Phases I and II. That's why Phase III also continues my mixture of old-school lifts, where you anchor your feet and lift as much as you can; along with more functional training on unstable surfaces. The Bosu ball pushup

HEY, MARIO!

I'm trying to shed pounds, but I'm friggin' tired of eating bananas, oranges, and apples. What's another healthy fruit?

Have you tried grapefruit? In a study done at Scripps Institute, subjects who ate half of one three times a day lost significantly more weight than folks in a group that didn't. That was the only variable, too—all they did was eat grapefruit. The egg-heads aren't sure why, but grapefruit seems to enhance metabolism while helping to control insulin.

9 WAYS TO JUMPSTART YOUR WORKOUTS

1) "Pre-exhaust" your muscles. When most people lift weights, they do the biggest move for a body part first, followed by the smaller moves. The problem comes when, say, you start off your back workout with barbell rows, only to feel your biceps fail first, not your lats. Pre-exhaustion fakes out that limitation. Kick off your back workout with a smaller, more isolated move—such as a straight-arm pulldown—and *then* do the bigger move, such as a barbell row. Now, with your back fatigued but your biceps fresh as daisies, obliterate your lats. Other pre-exhaustion combinations I like include cable flys before bench presses, and leg extensions before squats.

2) Confuse your muscle groups. The moment muscles grow accustomed to a move, kiss progress good-bye. That's why I never perform two identical workouts for a particular muscle group. You don't need to reinvent the wheel every time out, but simple changes like using a different cable attachment every time you do lat pulldowns will keep your muscles guessing and growing.

3) Circuit train. Once you've mastered your routine, it's time to kick up the pace and reorder your workout, making speed a priority. Instead of finishing each stage of a six- or seven-exercise routine in order, go from station to station, doing one set of each exercise. Give yourself two to three minutes in between each circuit and go through it again, repeating it until you've completed three to four rounds. It's an exhausting technique, but well worth the effort.

4) Keep a log. In my experience, taking mental notes on my physical progress has never been that effective. But I have benefited greatly from writing down every set, every rep, and the weights I used in a notebook. It helps me track my development. As we've already discussed, the second layer of this is writing down what you eat and tallying your daily caloric intake. You'll be less likely to splurge on dessert when you know you have to own up to it in your log.

5) Change the mix. Sometimes, getting that extra adrenalin boost is as simple as hearing a new tune with some giddy-up. Whatever your musical tastes, the link between upbeat music and physical energy cannot be denied. If you don't listen to music when you work out, I highly recommend making the investment in an iPod. Or, you could try altering other stimuli. If you typically get most of your exercising done inside a gym, take it outside and let the sun and wind breathe new life into you. You'll find great ways to do that scattered throughout this book.

6) Find a partner. I would have never made it very far in the gym—or anywhere else in life—without the fire burning deep within myself. But a lifting partner with similar goals can help push you to the next level with their advice, example, and encouragement. Choose your partner wisely, though. A chatterbox can smother an otherwise effective workout.

7) Take a class. Spin routines or aerobic rooms with instructors take the partner effect and multiply it tenfold. I used to think I was pushing myself hard in my solo workouts—and I was—but there's really no accounting for how hard you can work in a room crowded with people doing the same exercise. If aerobics and spin classes aren't your thing, take a shot at Tae Bo or boxing lessons. It really doesn't matter what discipline you choose, as long as the intensity can spike your cardio levels.

8) Accentuate the negative. Slow down the negative part of a movement until you almost can't take it any more. For example: Step into the squat rack with a weight that normally allows you to complete 10 to 15 reps with no problem. Now control the squat with a 10-second negative . . . and feel your muscles yelp for mercy. Applying this technique to virtually any exercise will increase strength and size.

9) Weed out the weak. A body part that clearly isn't on par with the rest of your physique, needs some extra attention that it hasn't been receiving. Sometimes, I start by working what I consider my weak links first. This way, the weaker muscles are worked when I have the most energy, and they can start to catch up with the rest of my body.

exemplifies the latter. Turn it upside down, grasp the sides with your hands, and rep from that position. Not only are you working what you would expect to work—chest and triceps—but your core will face a major gut check to help you complete the lift. Researchers at the University of Minnesota found that unstable pushups recruited the serratus anterior—the ribbed muscle that fans up from the ribs to the shoulder blades—38 percent more than your basic pushup does. This pays big dividends in the boxing ring; in fact, some people call the serratus anterior "the boxer's muscle." When you throw a punch, the serratus is one reason you can draw back that shoulder blade and thrust forward with a punch. It'll also help when you twist to reach a shot during a game of beach volleyball.

My desire to perfect your entire core explains why you'll be doing crunches on a Swiss ball, rather than flat on the floor. Using the Swiss ball is a good way to generate additional oblique activity because the surface gives, and it's a little unstable. The oblique muscles angle up and away from the sides of your abdominals. (Put your hands in your pockets. Your forearms now shadow your obliques.) Like the serratus, the obliques are smaller, less-used muscles. Yet they serve several crucial functions, including trunk rotation. You can imagine how important that is when dancing, boxing, playing basketball, and twisting into the yoga positions described in Chapter 5.

Regardless of the exercise you're about to do, make sure to read my written descriptions accompanying the photographs. These how-tos include technique suggestions and subtle tips that can make a huge difference in a move's effectiveness.

PHASE III PRIMARY GOALS:

- Improved strength
- Greater power
- Improved body composition

Phase III

Beginners							
	Monday	Tuesday	Wednesday	Thursday	Friday	Saturday	Sunday
WEEK 1:	Workout A	Rest	Workout B	Rest	Workout C	Workout D	Rest
WEEK 2:	Workout A	Rest	Workout B	Rest	Workout C	Workout F	Rest
WEEK 3:	Workout A	Rest	Workout B	Rest	Workout C	Workout D	Rest
WEEK 4:	Workout A	Rest	Workout B	Rest	Workout C	Workout F	Rest
Intermediates and Advanced							
	Monday	Tuesday	Wednesday	Thursday	Friday	Saturday	Sunday
WEEK 1:	Workout A	Rest	Workout B	Workout D	Workout C	Workout F	Rest
WEEK 2:	Workout A	Rest	Workout B	Workout D	Workout C	Workout F	Rest

Phase III:
Workout A

Sequence	Week	Exercise	Sets[1]	Reps[2]	Rest[3]
A1	1	Squat/Push Press	3	12–15	↑30
	2	Squat/Push Press	3	12–15	↑30
	3	Squat/Push Press	3	12–15	↑30
	4	Squat/Push Press	3	12–15	↑30
A2	1	Dumbbell One-Arm Row	3	12–15/side	↑30
	2	Dumbbell One-Arm Row	3	12–15/side	↑30
	3	Dumbbell One-Arm Row	3	12–15/side	↑30
	4	Dumbbell One-Arm Row	3	12–15/side	↑30
A3	1	Dumbbell Swing	3	12–15	↑30
	2	Dumbbell Swing	3	12–15	↑30
	3	Dumbbell Swing	3	12–15	↑30
	4	Dumbbell Swing	3	12–15	↑30
A4	1	Bosu Ball Pushup	3	Up to 20	60
	2	Bosu Ball Pushup	3	Up to 20	60
	3	Bosu Ball Pushup	3	Up to 20	60
	4	Bosu Ball Pushup	3	Up to 20	60
B1	1	Incline Prone Dumbbell Y	3	12–15	↑30
	2	Incline Prone Dumbbell Y	3	12–15	↑30
	3	Incline Prone Dumbbell Y	3	12–15	↑30
	4	Incline Prone Dumbbell Y	3	12–15	↑30
B2	1	Pressdown	3	12–15	↑30
	2	Pressdown	3	12–15	↑30
	3	Pressdown	3	12–15	↑30
	4	Pressdown	3	12–15	↑30
B3	1	Seated Zottman Curl	3	12–15	↑30
	2	Seated Zottman Curl	3	12–15	↑30
	3	Seated Zottman Curl	3	12–15	↑30
	4	Seated Zottman Curl	3	12–15	↑30
B4	1	Swiss Ball Crunch	3	12–15	60
	2	Swiss Ball Crunch	3	12–15	60
	3	Swiss Ball Crunch	3	12–15	60
	4	Swiss Ball Crunch	3	12–15	60
C1		Perform treadmill intervals: Walk for 3 minutes at a easy pace, then perform 6–8 repetitions of 30-second sprints followed by 90 seconds of walking.			

[1] Do modified supersets with each pair of exercises listed with the same number (for example, A1 and A2); that is, do the prescribed number of sets for each of the two exercises in alternating fashion before moving on to the next pairing. (For example, if the program calls for three sets, do one set of split squats followed by one set of push-ups, and then repeat twice). Rest in between each set as prescribed.

[2] The last rep you can finish with complete control and perfect form should fall within this range, so select your weight accordingly. Once you have completed all your repetitions with your current weight for two consecutive workouts, increase your poundage slightly. Five pounds for each new step is a good rule of thumb.

[3] Between supersets, measured in seconds.

SQUAT/ PUSH PRESS

Great for:
volleyball,
raquetball

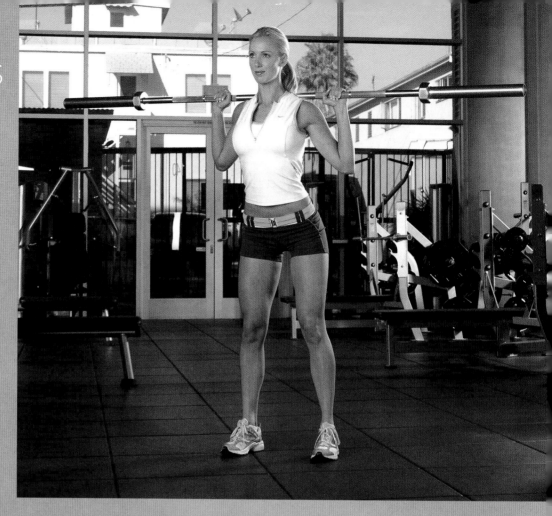

Get ready!

Stand with a barbell resting across your traps. Your chest should be up and out, and your abs should be tight.

Go!

Bend at the hips and knees to lower your body, descending until your thighs are parallel to the floor. As you return to the starting position, explosively press the barbell overhead. Lower the barbell back to its original position and sink into the next rep without hesitation.

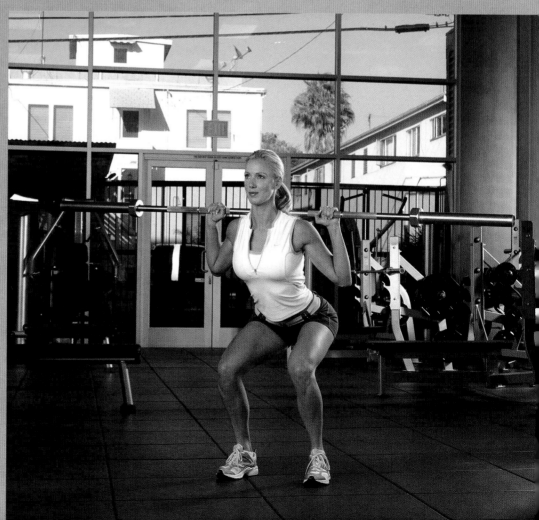

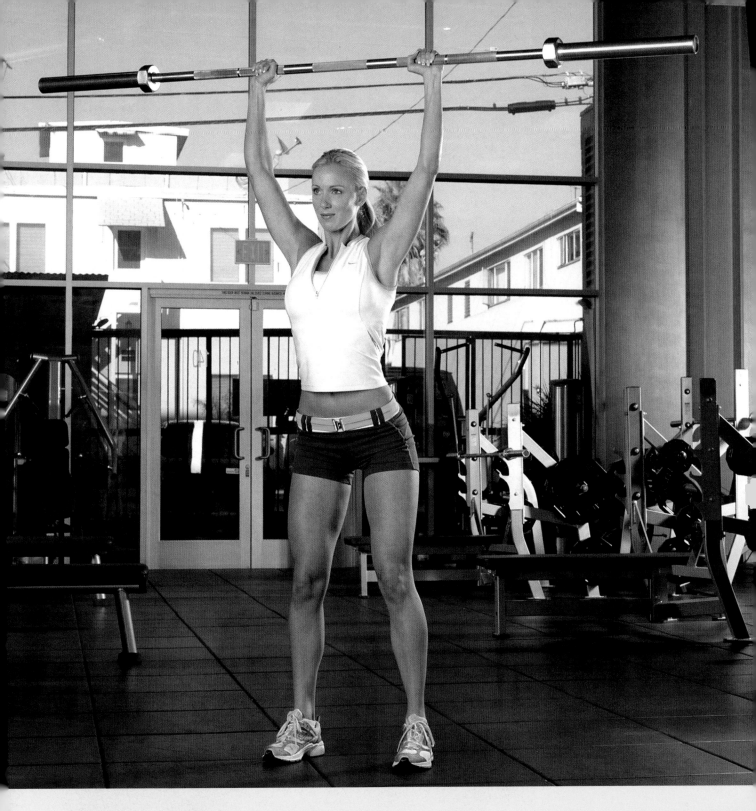

Watch out for:

Lack of explosiveness. As the name implies, a push press is different from a conventional press. Use your legs like springs to drive up the barbell. Also, watch out for your heels coming up off the floor during the squat portion of the lift. If they do, your calves are tight and will need to be stretched.

DUMBBELL ONE-ARM ROW

Great for: flag football, sailing

Get ready!

Holding a dumbbell in your left hand, place your right hand and right knee on a bench. Your torso should be bent forward about 90 degrees.

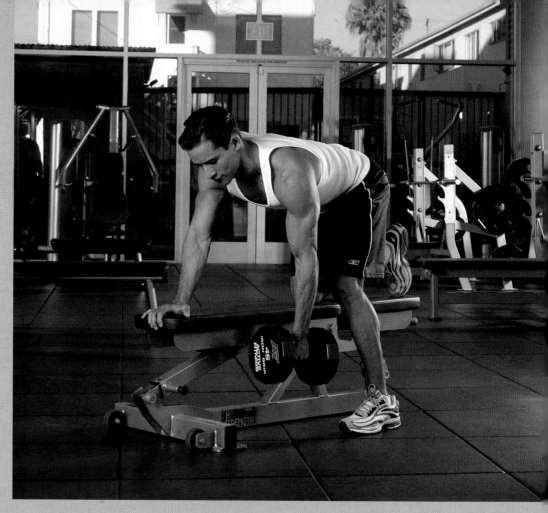

Go!

Hold the weight with your arm straight and just in front of your shoulder. Use your upper back muscles to pull the dumbbell up and back toward your hip. Pause, then slowly lower the weight.

Tweak:

Instead of kneeling on a bench, you can also grasp a dumbbell rack with one hand for support.

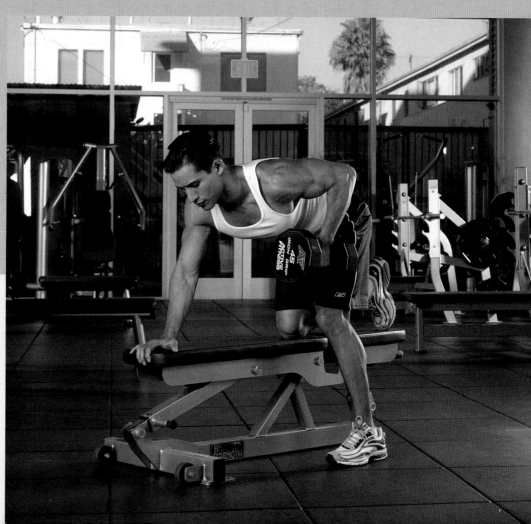

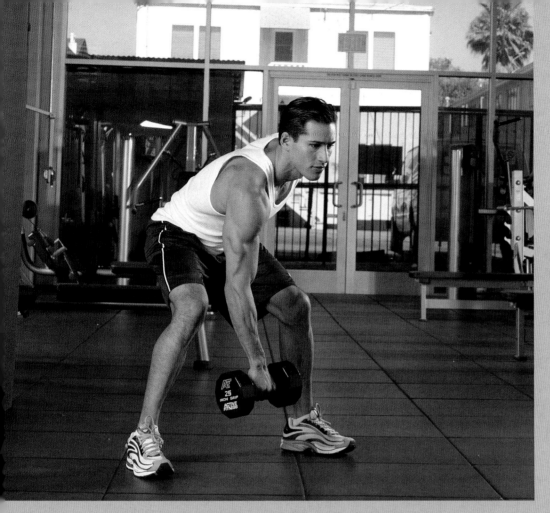

DUMBBELL SWING

Great for: track and field, football

Get ready!

Stand holding a dumbbell in your right hand with your feet just beyond shoulder-width apart. Push back your hips and bend your knees so that the weight hangs at arm's length between your legs, just above ankle height. Your torso will be angled forward but your back should be flat, not rounded.

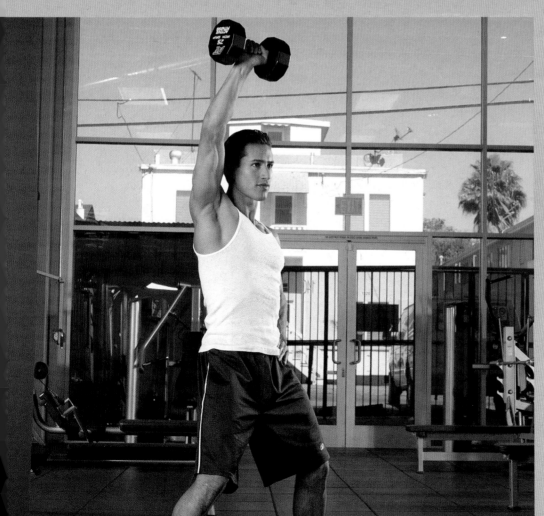

Go!

Explode out of your crouch, swinging the weight overhead as your hips and knees straighten. At the top, your arm should be fully extended overhead and your knees should have only a very slight bend in them.

BOSU BALL PUSHUP

Great for: surfing, rock climbing

Get ready!

Assume the standard pushup position, only your hands should grasp the sides of a Bosu ball that is upside down, deliberately making it unstable. Straighten your legs behind you so your body forms a straight line from head to heels.

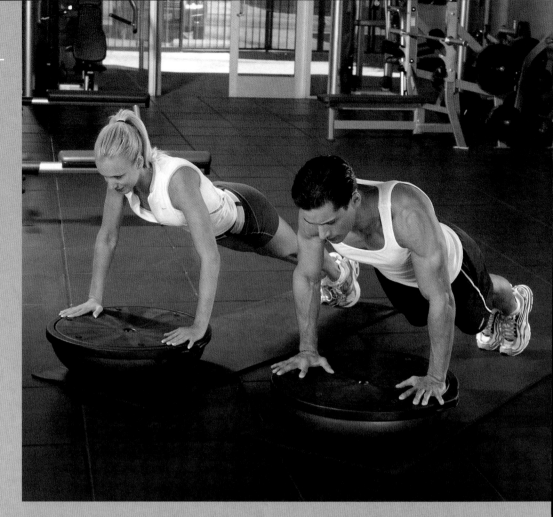

Go!

Bend your elbows to lower your torso until your chest is just off the floor. Push yourself back to the starting position.

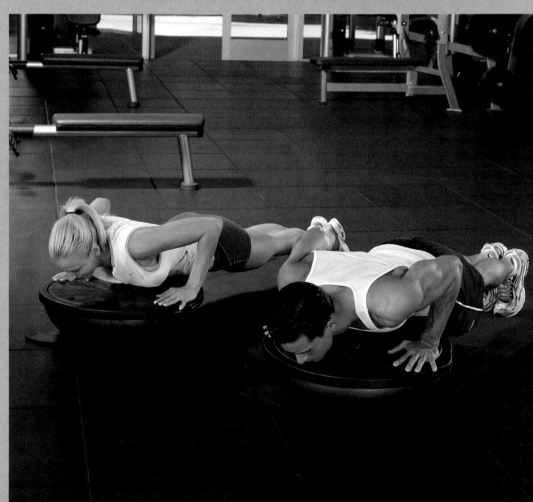

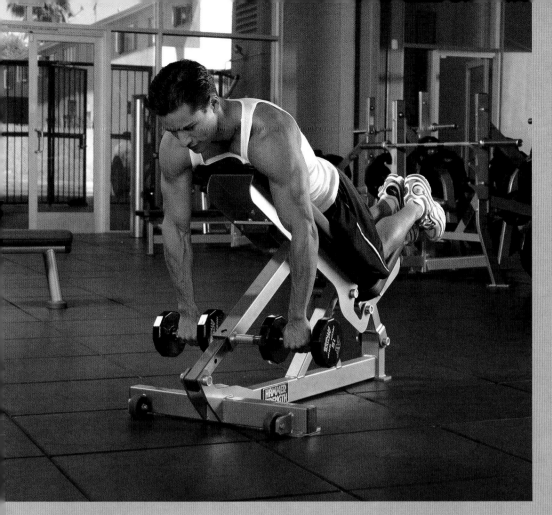

INCLINE PRONE DUMBBELL "Y"

Great for:
hang gliding, horseback riding

Get ready!

Lie facedown on an incline bench—ideally the angle should be 45 degrees—holding two dumbbells at arm's length.

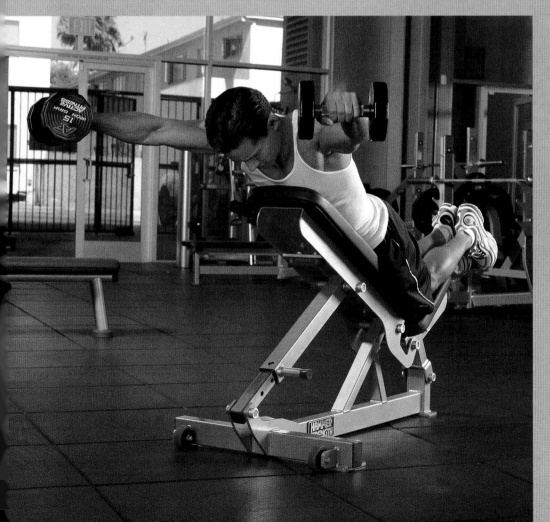

Go!

Keeping your elbows slightly bent but your wrists straight, slowly raise your arms straight out to form the shape of a Y. Return to the starting position.

PRESSDOWN

Great for: gymnastics, lacrosse

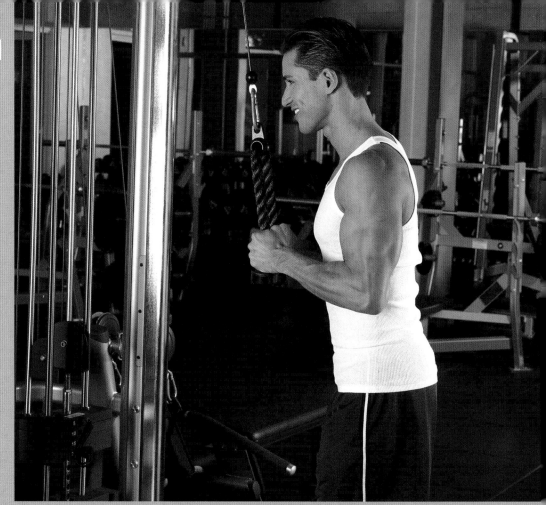

Get ready!

Stand in front of a cable stack, grasping a rope handle attached to the high pulley. To reach the start position, bring your elbows in close to your body and push down until your forearms are parallel with the floor.

Go!

Extend your elbows to press the handle down until it reaches the front of your thighs. Just before you reach lockout, pause for a quick triceps squeeze, and then resist the pull of the cable on the way back to the starting position.

Watch out for:

Cheating on your form by leaning forward to push down on the resistance with your whole body, not just your triceps. Lean forward only slightly. Better yet, don't lean at all!

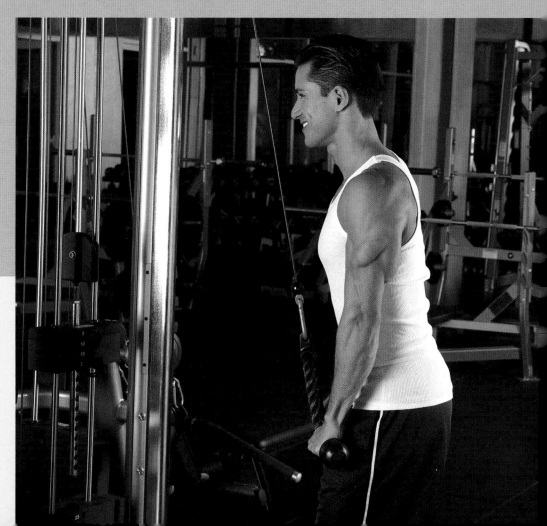

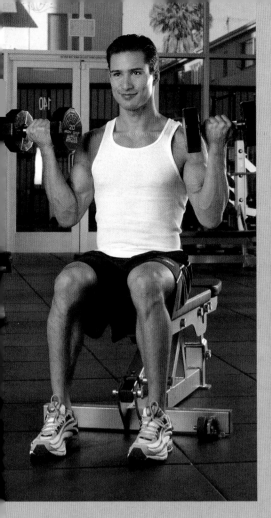
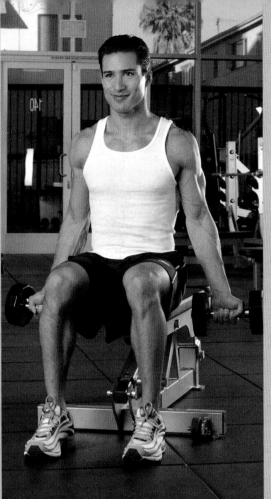
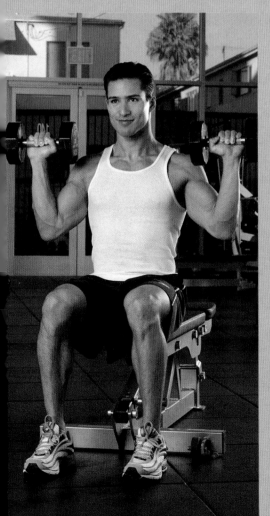
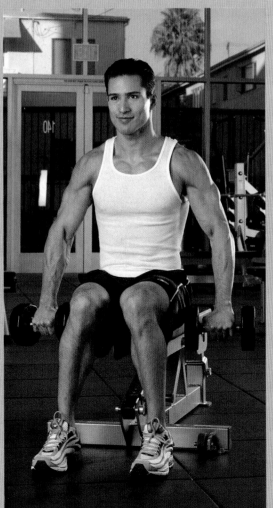

Great for:
hockey, bowling

Get ready!

Sit on a bench holding a pair of dumbbells so that your palms face behind you. Let the weights hang at arm's length at your sides.

Go!

Without moving your upper arms, curl the weights up toward your shoulders. At the top, rotate your wrists so your palms face forward. Lower the weights back to the starting position, rotating your wrists again near the bottom.

177

SWISS BALL CRUNCH

Great for:
skiing, cycling

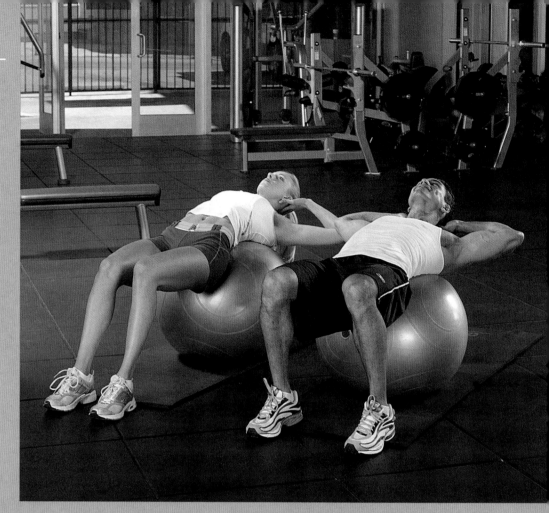

Get ready!

Lie on your back on a Swiss ball so that your lower back and hips rest on its surface. Place your fingertips behind your ears.

Go!

Raise your torso as high as you can by crunching your chest toward your hips. Lower back to the starting position, and repeat.

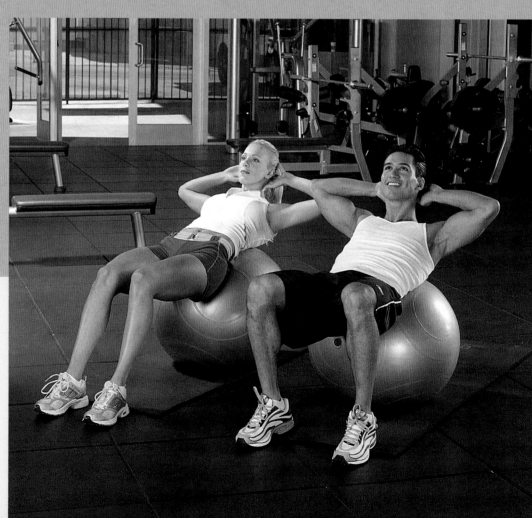

Tweaks:

If you don't feel like you're getting enough out of the move, make sure that only your lower back, not your shoulders, are on the ball.

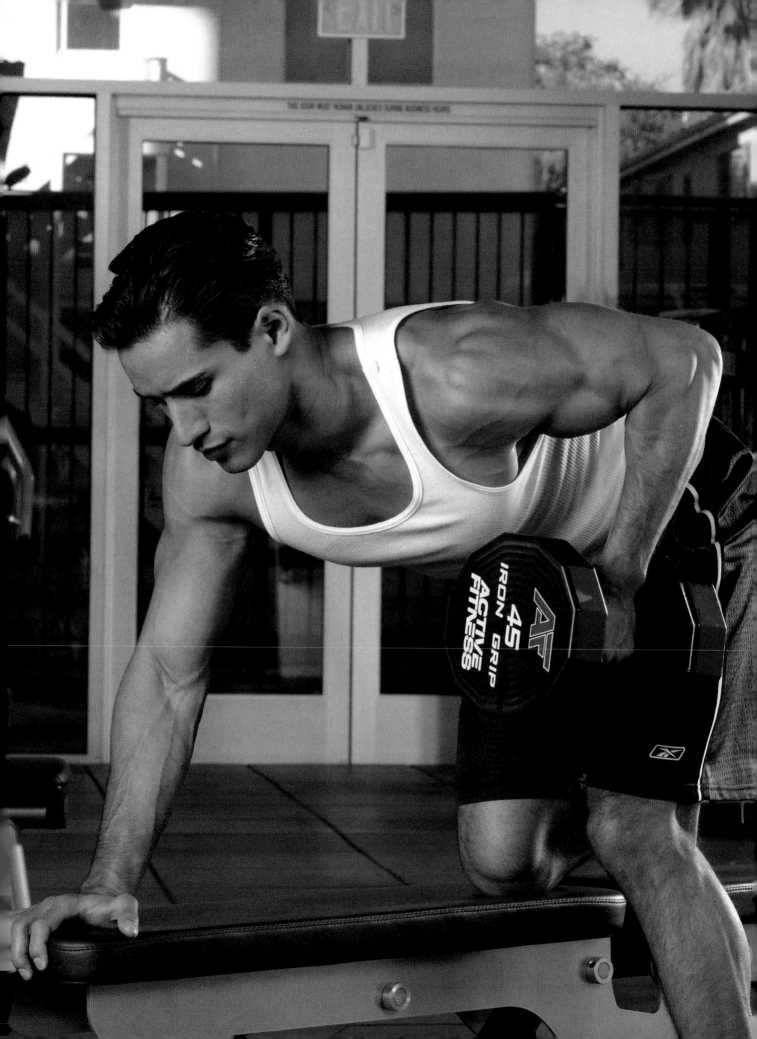

Phase III:
Workout B

Sequence	Week	Exercise	Sets[1]	Reps[2]	Rest[3]
A1	1	Deadlift	3	8–10	↑60
	1	Deadlift	3	8–10	↑60
	1	Deadlift	3	8–10	↑60
	1	Deadlift	3	8–10	↑60
A2	1	Flat-Bench Barbell Press	3	8–10	↑60
	1	Flat-Bench Barbell Press	3	8–10	↑60
	1	Flat-Bench Barbell Press	3	8–10	↑60
	1	Flat-Bench Barbell Press	3	8–10	↑60
B1	1	Swiss Ball Reverse Back Extension	3	8–10	↑60
	1	Swiss Ball Reverse Back Extension	3	8–10	↑60
	1	Swiss Ball Reverse Back Extension	3	8–10	↑60
	1	Swiss Ball Reverse Back Extension	3	8–10	↑60
B2	1	Standing Two-Arm Cable Row	3	8–10/side	↑60
	1	Standing Two-Arm Cable Row	3	8–10/side	↑60
	1	Standing Two-Arm Cable Row	3	8–10/side	↑60
	1	Standing Two-Arm Cable Row	3	8–10/side	↑60
C1	1	Barbell Push Press	3	8–10	↑60
	2	Barbell Push Press	3	8–10	↑60
	3	Barbell Push Press	3	8–10	↑60
	4	Barbell Push Press	3	8–10	↑60
C2	1	Standing Cable Curl	3	8–10	↑60
	1	Standing Cable Curl	3	8–10	↑60
	1	Standing Cable Curl	3	8–10	↑60
	1	Standing Cable Curl	3	8–10	↑60
D1	1	Russian Twist	3	8–10/side	↑60
	1	Russian Twist	3	8–10/side	↑60
	1	Russian Twist	3	8–10/side	↑60
	1	Russian Twist	3	8–10/side	↑60
E1		Perform treadmill intervals: Walk for 3 minutes at a easy pace, then perform 5–6 repetitions of 60-second sprints followed by 120 seconds of walking.			

[1] Do modified supersets with each pair of exercises listed with the same number (for example, A1 and A2); that is, do the prescribed number of sets for each of the two exercises in alternating fashion before moving on to the next pairing. (For example, if the program calls for three sets, do one set of split squats followed by one set of push-ups, and then repeat twice). Rest in between each set as prescribed.

[2] The last rep you can finish with complete control and perfect form should fall within this range, so select your weight accordingly. Once you have completed all your repetitions with your current weight for two consecutive workouts, increase your poundage slightly. Five pounds for each new step is a good rule of thumb.

[3] Between supersets, measured in seconds.

DEADLIFT

Great for: football, martial arts

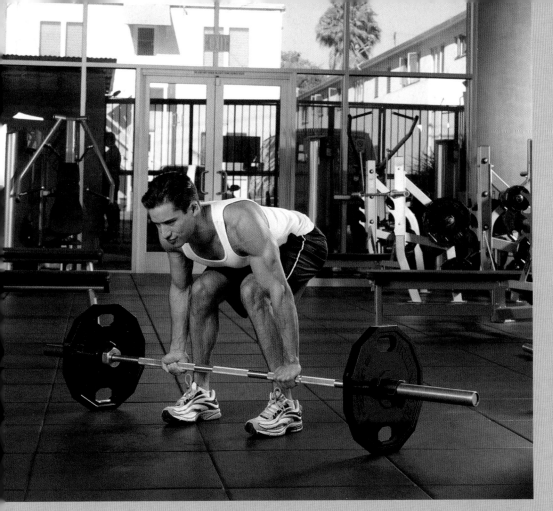

Get ready!

Stand in front of a barbell on the floor so that your shins touch the bar. Bend your knees and grasp the bar with one hand overhand and one hand under-hand. Your elbows should be just out-side your knees.

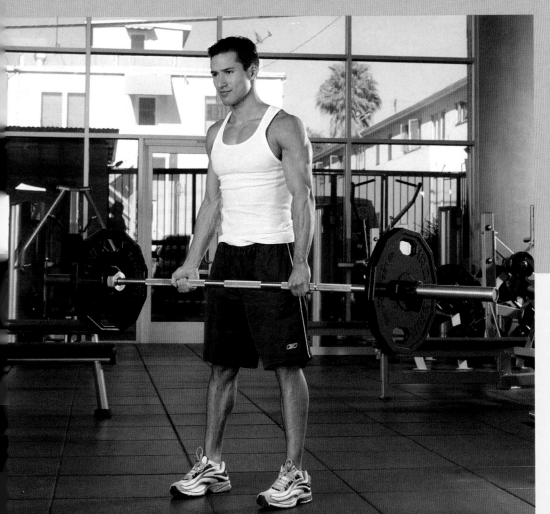

Go!

Keeping your head and back straight, stand up by pressing through the floor with your legs and dragging the bar up your thighs. Pause to squeeze your legs and glutes, and then slowly lower the bar.

Watch our for:

Bar drift. Keep the weight as close to your body as pos-sible throughout the entire lift.

FLAT-BENCH BARBELL PRESS

Great for:
wrestling, rugby

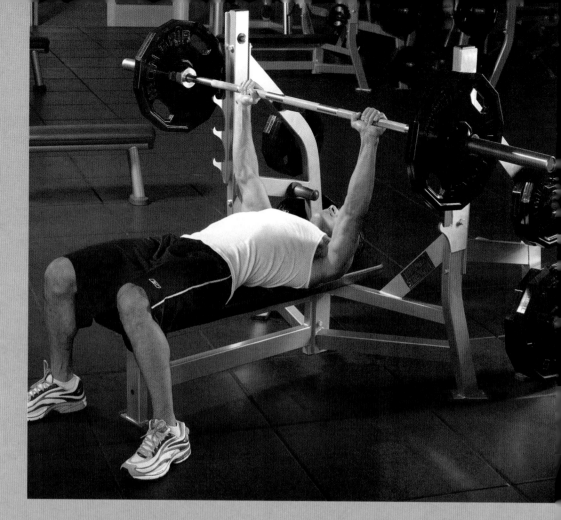

Get ready!

Lie face-up with your back flat against the pad. Grasp the bar with both hands, take it off the rack, and raise it to arm's length above you.

Go!

Lower the bar at a three-count until it touches your chest. Without "bouncing" off the bottom, push the weight back up at a two-count to the starting position.

Watch out for:

Losing control of the bar. This is one exercise where you definitely want an attentive spotter on hand at all times.

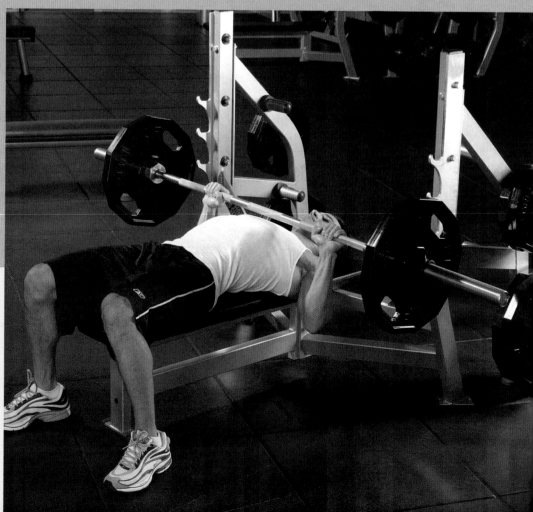

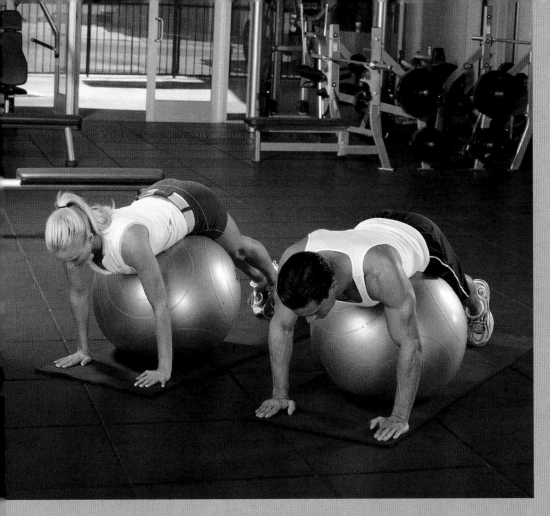

SWISS BALL REVERSE BACK EXTENSION

Great for:
soccer, swimming

Get ready!

Lie facing down on a Swiss ball so that your torso and hips are in contact with the surface of the ball. Your legs should extend behind you so your toes touch the floor. Your hands should be touching the ground for balance.

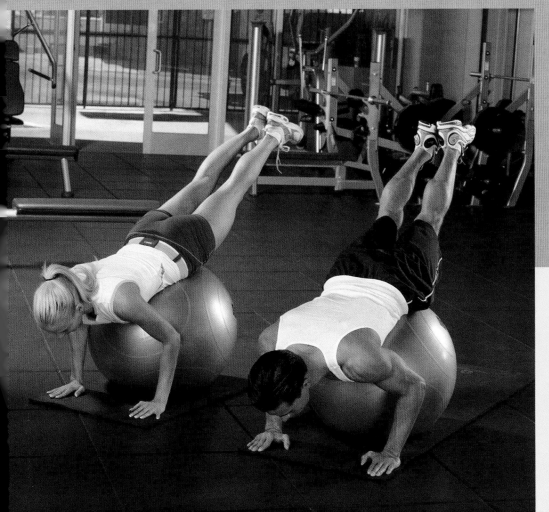

Go!

Raise your legs until they extend directly behind you. Your body should form a straight line at this point.

Watch out for:

Hyperextension at the top of the movement, which is bad. This occurs when your legs come up so high that your body moves past a straight line.

183

STANDING TWO-ARM CABLE ROW

Great for:
wrestling, climbing

Get ready!

Attach a "V" handle to a low cable pulley. Grab the handle with both hands and stand back a few feet from the weight stack. Bend at the knees and hips, so that your torso is angled forward slightly.

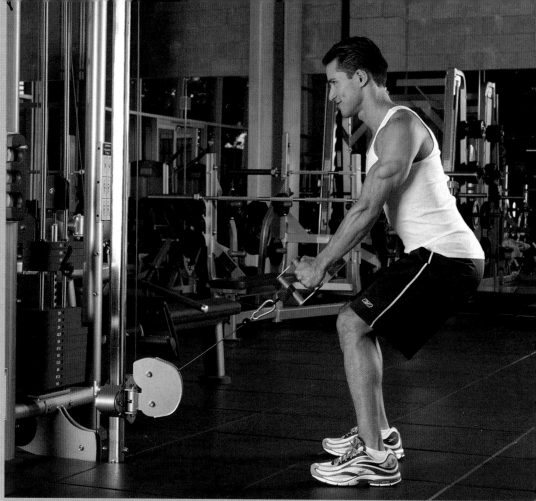

Go!

Row the handle toward your upper abs until your elbows pass your torso, then resist the weight as your arms straighten back out in front of you.

Watch out for:

A rounded back. Keeping your chest up and your shoulders back should help keep your spine in its natural position.

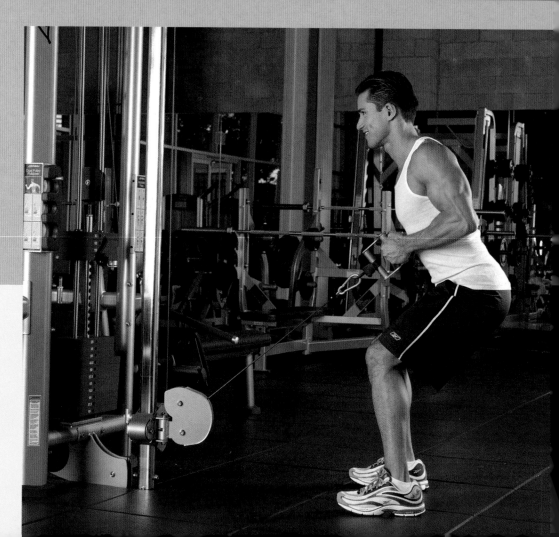
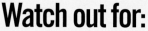

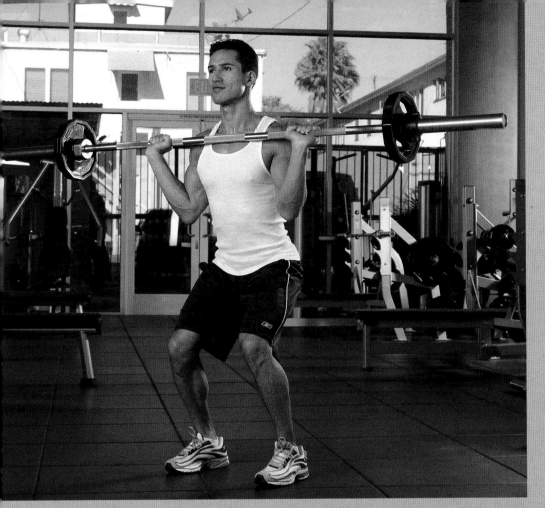

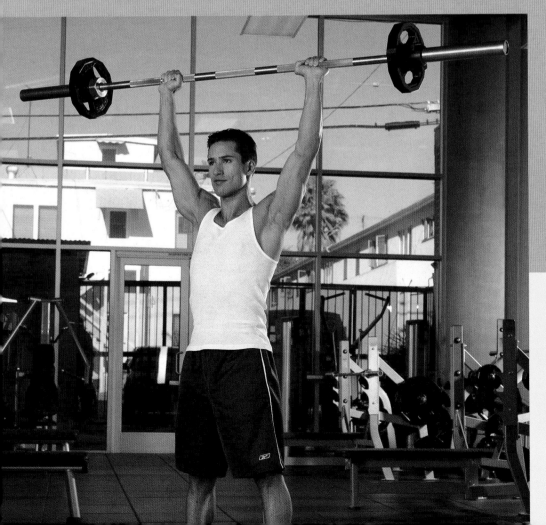

BARBELL PUSH PRESS

Great for:
volleyball,
basketball

Get ready!

Stand holding a barbell across your shoulder girdle using an overhand grip, hands slightly wider than shoulder-width apart.

Go!

Bend your knees to descend very slightly—say, six inches—and then immediately use your legs to drive up, pushing the bar overhead. Return to the starting position.

Watch out for:

Arching your back to help lift the bar overhead. Arching places potentially injury-producing pressure on the spine.

185

STANDING CABLE CURL

Great for:
horseback riding, baseball

Get ready!

Stand facing a cable stack holding an EZ curl bar attachment at arm's length using a shoulder-width underhand grip.

Go!

Bend your elbows to raise the bar until the handle reaches shoulder level. Return to the starting position.

Watch out for:

Back sensation. If you feel this move there, you're using body momentum, which means you're not focusing the move enough on your biceps.

186

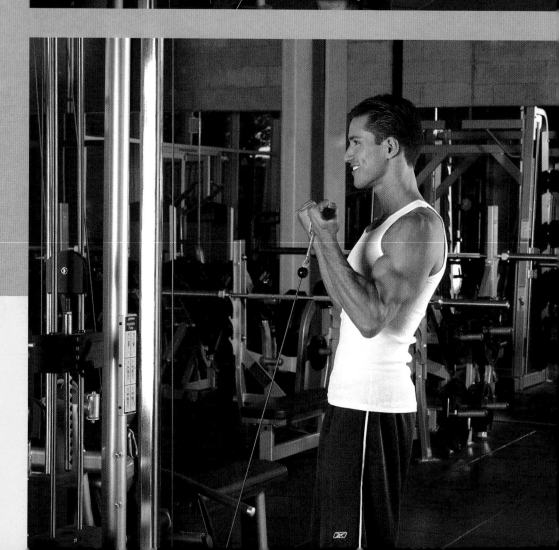

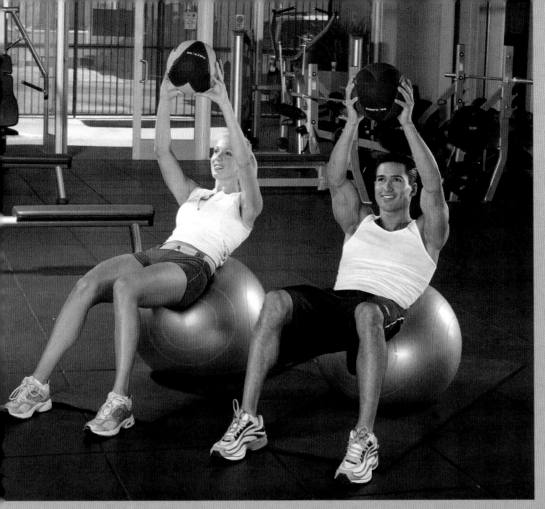

RUSSIAN TWIST

Great for:
tennis, golf

Get ready!

Lie facing up on a Swiss ball, and hold a dumbbell or medicine ball overhead with both hands.

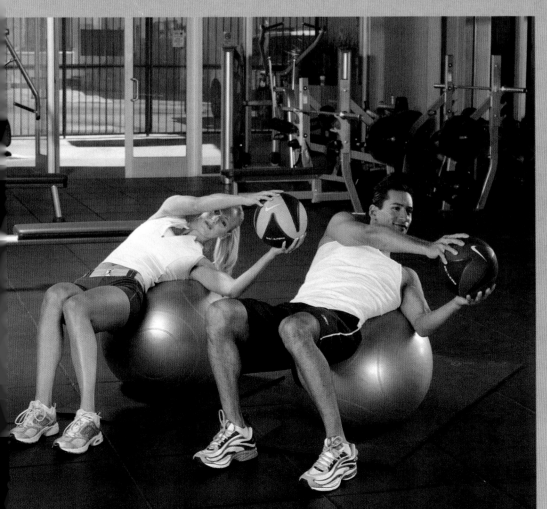

Go!

Keeping your arms straight, rotate your torso to bring the weight down until your arms have gone from being perpendicular to the floor to parallel. Rotate back to the starting position, and then repeat the move, only to the other side. Continue alternating.

Phase III:
Workout C

Sequence	Week	Exercise	Sets[1]	Reps[2]	Rest[t]
A1	1	Front Squat	3	10–12	↑60
	2	Front Squat	3	10–12	↑60
	3	Front Squat	3	10–12	↑60
	4	Front Squat	3	10–12	↑60
A2	1	Bench Jump	3	4–6	↑90
	2	Bench Jump	3	4–6	↑90
	3	Bench Jump	3	4–6	↑90
	4	Bench Jump	3	4–6	↑90
B1	1	Incline Neutral-Grip Dumbbell Press	3	10–12	↑60
	2	Incline Neutral-Grip Dumbbell Press	3	10–12	↑60
	3	Incline Neutral-Grip Dumbbell Press	3	10–12	↑60
	4	Incline Neutral-Grip Dumbbell Press	3	10–12	↑60
B2	1	Medicine Ball Toss	3	6–8	↑90
	2	Medicine Ball Toss	3	6–8	↑90
	3	Medicine Ball Toss	3	6–8	↑90
	4	Medicine Ball Toss	3	6–8	↑90
C1	1	Chinup	3	10–12	↑60
	2	Chinup	3	10–12	↑60
	3	Chinup	3	10–12	↑60
	4	Chinup	3	10–12	↑60
C2	1	Medicine Ball Overhead Throw	3	6–8	↑90
	2	Medicine Ball Overhead Throw	3	6–8	↑90
	3	Medicine Ball Overhead Throw	3	6–8	↑90
	4	Medicine Ball Overhead Throw	3	6–8	↑90
D1	1	Swiss Ball Knee Tuck	3	10–12	↑60
	2	Swiss Ball Knee Tuck	3	10–12	↑60
	3	Swiss Ball Knee Tuck	3	10–12	↑60
	4	Swiss Ball Knee Tuck	3	10–12	↑60
E1		Perform treadmill intervals: Walk for 3 minutes at a easy pace, then perform 4–6 repetitions of 90–120-second sprints followed by 120 seconds of walking.			

[1] Do modified supersets with each pair of exercises listed with the same number (for example, A1 and A2); that is, do the prescribed number of sets for each of the two exercises in alternating fashion before moving on to the next pairing. (For example, if the program calls for three sets, do one set of split squats followed by one set of push-ups, and then repeat twice). Rest in between each set as prescribed.

[2] The last rep you can finish with complete control and perfect form should fall within this range, so select your weight accordingly. Once you have completed all your repetitions with your current weight for two consecutive workouts, increase your poundage slightly. Five pounds for each new step is a good rule of thumb.

[3] Between supersets, measured in seconds.

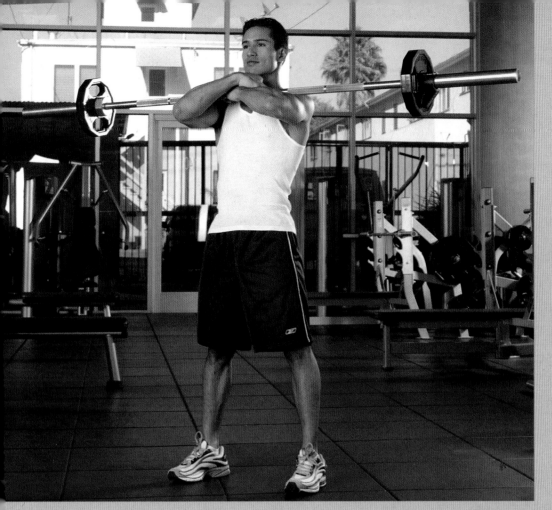

FRONT SQUAT

Great for: football, track and field

Get ready!

Hold a bar across your shoulder girdle so that your arms and hands are crossed in front of you on top of the bar. Set your feet shoulder-width apart and keep your back straight.

Go!

Without changing the position of your arms, lower your body until your thighs are parallel to the floor. Return to the starting position.

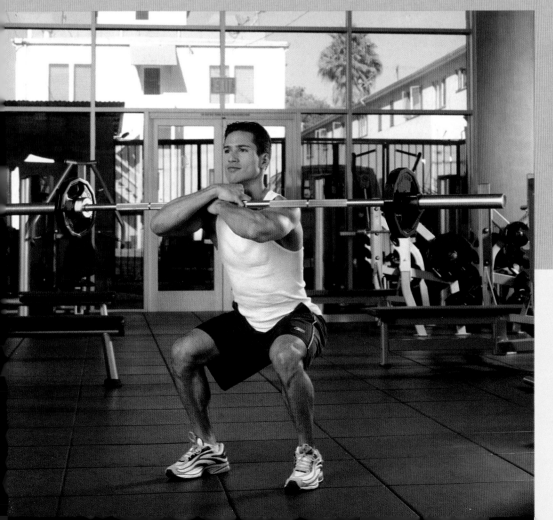

Watch out for:

The tendency to look up. Focus your eyes straight ahead throughout the move.

BENCH JUMP

Great for: track and field, basketball

Get ready!

Stand in front of a bench.

Go!

Bend at the knees and waist to jump explosively onto the bench's surface, which should be about knee high. Immediately jump backward, absorbing the impact by descending into a crouch and swinging your arms behind your body. Jump back and forth as fast as possible until completing the reps. The less time you spend on the floor or the bench, the better, but never lose your balance.

Caution:

Missing a jump can lead to serious injury. Before you jump, step on the bench to get a sense of its height. Also, end your set before you become totally fatigued. If your form becomes sloppy, injury could result.

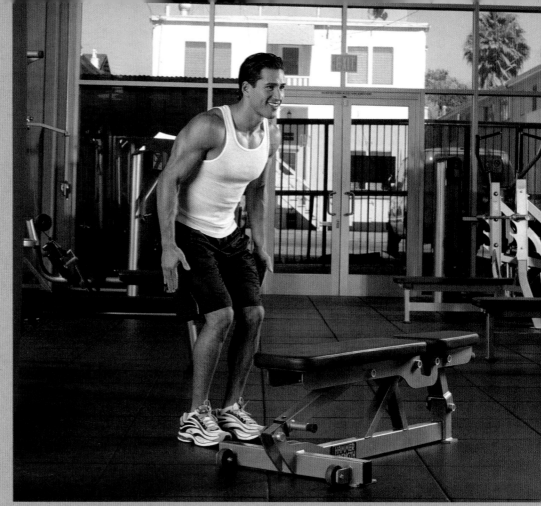

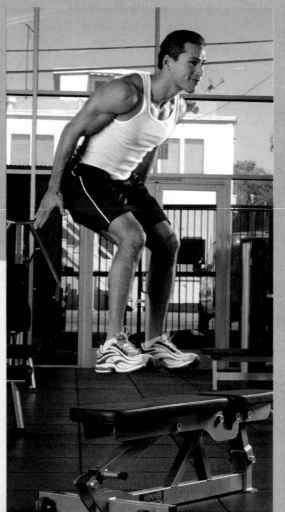

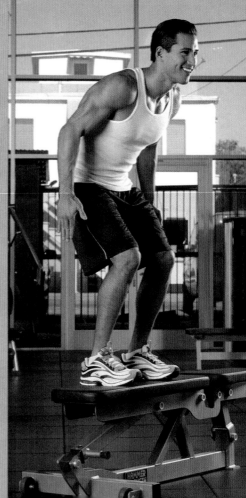

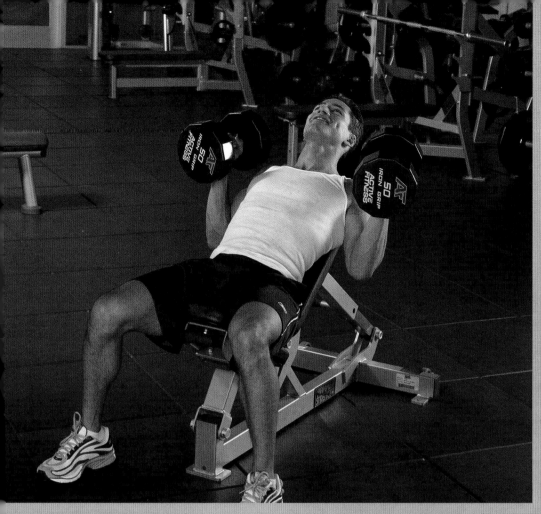

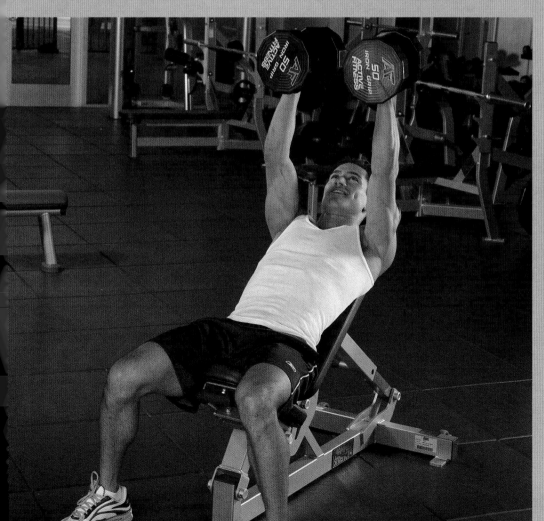

INCLINE NEUTRAL-GRIP DUMBBELL PRESS

Great for:
boxing, baseball

Get ready!

Grab a pair of dumbbells and lie on a bench facing up. Your grip should be neutral, meaning your palms face each other, not forward. Place your feet flat on the floor, draw in your abs, and push your lower back into the pad.

Go!

Press the dumbbells above you in a slightly arching line toward the midline of your chest. It's not necessary to clank the weights together—1 to 2 inches should separate them. Squeeze your chest muscles at the top of the move. Then reverse the same arching motion to lower the dumbbells back down in a controlled motion.

MEDICINE BALL CHEST TOSS

Great for: basketball, football

Get ready!

Find a place in the gym with open space in front of you, where a partner can stand awaiting your toss. Stand holding a medicine ball—up to 16 pounds for guys, up to 8 pounds for women—in front of your chest. Flare your elbows out to the sides, as if you are about to throw a classic basketball chest pass.

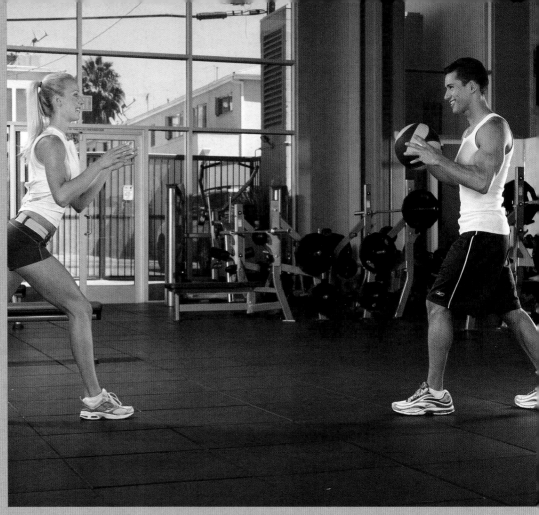

Go!

Pass it to your partner. Once it's returned, begin your second rep, and continue in alternating fashion.

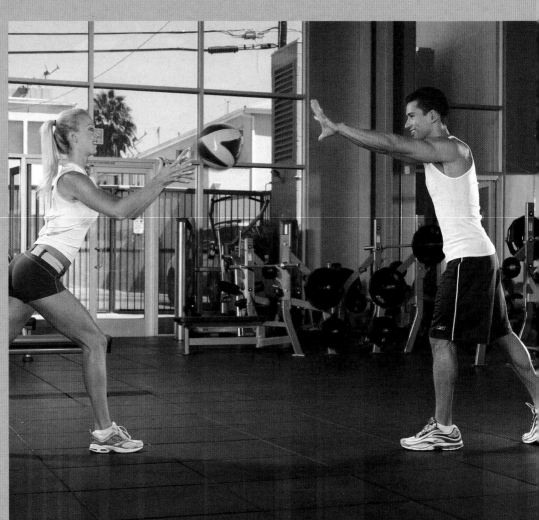

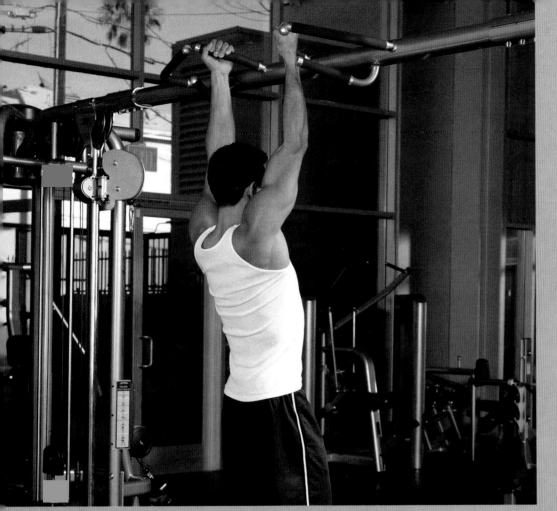

Great for:
rock climbing,
track and field

Get ready!

Grab a chinup bar
or handles with an
underhand grip,
hands spaced about
a foot apart. Hang
with your arms
straight.

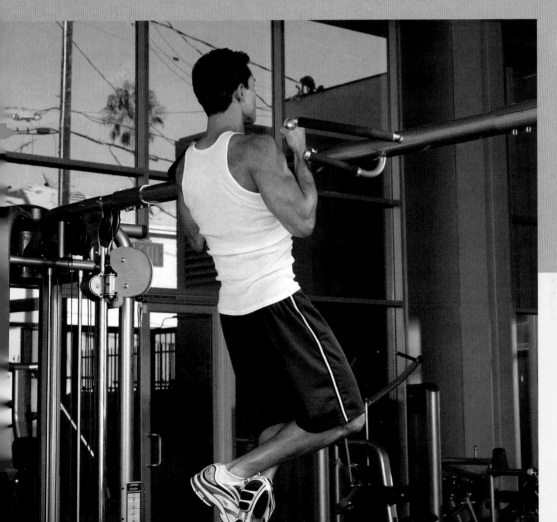

Go!

Keeping your head
straight and your
elbows pointed
down, pull yourself
up until the bar or
handles are directly
under your chin.
Then lower back to
the starting position.

Tweak:

If your body weight
is too much for you
to pull up, place a
chair or bench under
the bar to support
your feet.

193

MEDICINE BALL OVERHEAD THROW

Great for:
soccer, volleyball

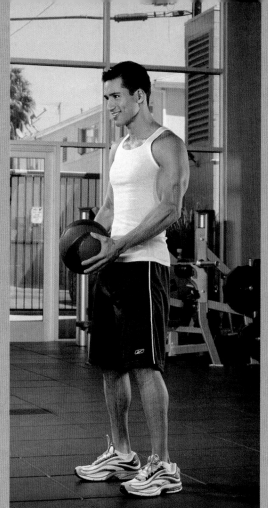
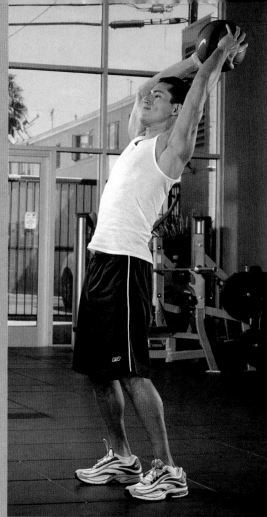

Get ready!

Stand holding a medicine ball—up to 16 pounds for guys, up to 8 pounds for women—at your waist.

Go!

Raise the ball over and behind your head.

Without stopping, throw the ball downward with both hands, so that it hits the ground 2 to 3 feet in front of you. Retrieve the ball and return to the starting position for another rep.

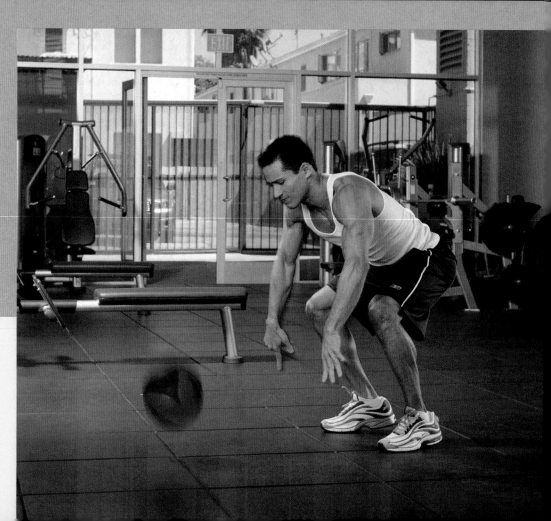

Tweak:

Medicine balls filled with sand work great for this move.

194

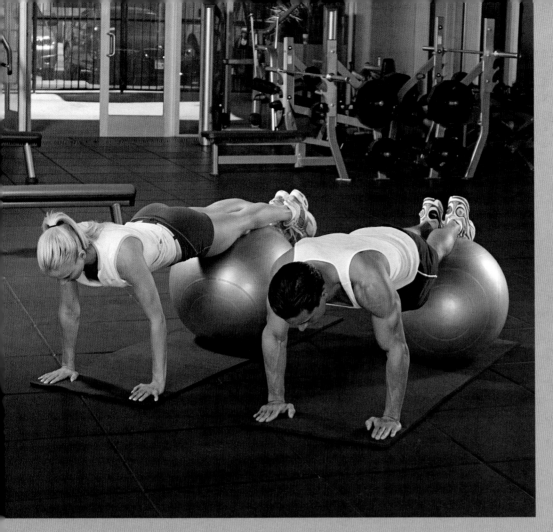

Get ready!

Assume a pushup position with your shins on top of a Swiss ball, hands spaced slightly wider than shoulder-width apart.

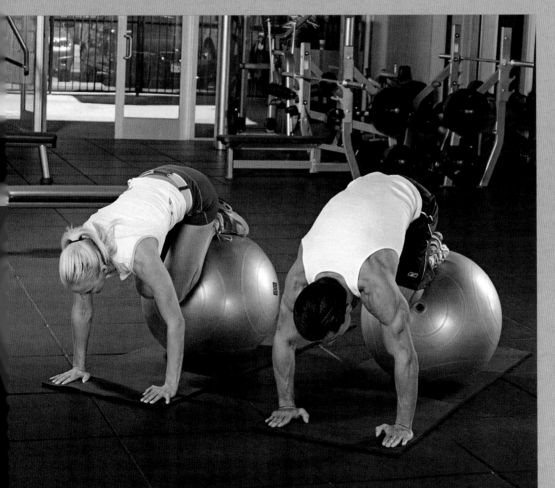

Go!

Keeping your abs tight, draw your knees toward your chest until your toes touch the top of the ball. Slowly straighten your legs so the ball rolls back to the starting position.

Phase III:
Workout D
STEP UP:
MY DANCE WORKOUT

When I box, I dance around the ring. After competing on *Dancing with the Stars*, I know what it's like to dance around on a stage, too, with tens of millions of viewers watching your every step and misstep. No pressure there, huh?

Here's a news flash: Dancing is as hard as any sport you've ever tried in your life. If you've never done it, you're in for a shock.

Ballroom dancing also teaches us more about anatomy than we ever learned in science class. It reveals the existence of muscles you never even knew you had in your body. That's because you never use them—until, that is, you find yourself carrying your partner, a full-grown adult, around a dance floor. She's resting her weight on you, and you have to move both bodies—yours and hers—while struggling to maintain perfect posture.

It wasn't just a matter of being sore after rehearsal. The sport's effect on leg development is self-evident, if you've ever watched the show, but you'd be surprised at how well developed my back, neck, and shoulders became over the course of a mere four weeks practicing for *Dancing with the Stars*.

My partner, Karina Smirnoff, is an amazing artist on stage and wonderful person off it. Born in Kharkiv, Ukraine, she went on to become the U.S. National Champion in ballroom dancing on five separate occasions. Now, she travels the world to teach dance. She's got a great body; she's built like a fighter. Through her eyes, I too fell in love with the ballroom dancing world, appreciating it not only as an art form but also as an unbelievably effective workout. Dancing can sculpt you as much as pumping iron does. "And it's really fun," adds Karina. "Not only is it a great workout, but it also makes you think with both hemispheres of your brain. You're not just standing there doing some repetitive motion."

I'm going to let Karina, the expert, explain the physical attributes of a great dancer. "First, you need a lot of stamina," she says. "You also need overall control of your muscles. If you have some muscle groups that are weaker than others, you're probably going to struggle with tension. Stability is also really important. If you don't have good balance, you're going to fall over."

Balanced development . . . muscle control . . . stability . . . balance. Sound familiar? The characteristics outlined by Karina as ideal are the same ones embedded throughout all of my workouts, from the gym to the boxing ring.

No wonder champion dancers such as Karina hit the gym all the time. "I do work out," she says. "I do cardiovascular training and total-body workouts with weights. But dancing itself is still the best workout for me because it engages every muscle group in my body." What's the net result of combining dance workouts with cardio and full-body resistance workouts? "You don't get pumped; you become toned, with great posture and flexibility," she says. "You get muscles that are long, strong, and flexible. Sometimes when we dance, we wear those skimpy outfits, so you want to make sure that looks good."

No argument here. I'm sure America will second that.

Your posture is the first thing that will undergo a transformation from dance. You can't dance and twist if you're all curled up into a ball. The more you stretch upward and the more you lengthen your spine, the more flexible your midsection becomes. Posture is the single biggest difference between boxing and dance, as Karina found the season after I appeared, when her dance partner was Floyd Mayweather Jr., arguably the best boxer, pound for pound, on earth. He's won belts in five different weight classes.

"Floyd was five-foot-eight to begin with, but when he danced, his natural tendency was to crouch," says Karina. "So he literally became half my size. I was looking down at him all the time, and I was like, 'You've got to straighten up!' He's got amazing footwork, and he can lean back like a character in *The Matrix* because he has such an incredibly strong core. But in ballroom dancing, at a certain point, you've just got to stand tall and let people appreciate that you have the posture, that you're able to do it."

Many of the moves included in my workout program are great for dancing *and* posture. All those moves done on a Swiss ball, where you have to tighten your core while moving the weight? Perfect. Anything where your torso rotates from side to side as you hold either a ball or a handle attached to a cable and weight stack? Good for dancing, big time. Squats and lunges are great, too. If you think the former are only for meatheads, or that they'll bulk up your butt and thighs, think again. Karina does squats, and look at her body!

HEY, MARIO!

I enjoy drinking a glass of wine or two in the evening, especially after a hard day. Do I have to give up my vino on your program?

As long as you don't abuse it, keep drinking wine, red especially. It contains few carbohydrates, so it's perfect for evening consumption. It's also loaded with plant chemicals that scientists claim are responsible for all sorts of health benefits, from reducing the risk of heart disease and obesity to lowering the chances you'll be diagnosed with cancer.

As for the fat-burning potential of dance, just watch *Dancing with the Stars*. Every single celebrity loses flab, even those who were in good shape beforehand, like me. Heck, Joey Fatone, the actor and singer formerly with 'N Sync, lost 20 pounds in a matter of weeks!

I don't dance competitively any longer, like I did on the show, but I still do it for fun, and the whole experience remains a part of me. When I go to a hospital to visit sick children, dancing provides a great means of connecting with them. Just the other day, I visited an inner-city school in Las Vegas, and things really got rolling only after I pulled a kid from the audience and started dancing with her.

Karina has chosen the following six steps in part because they hit the whole body (although she singles out the area or areas of emphasis under each exercise name). All of these moves offer the experience of dancing plus a great workout. In fact, these are the steps I danced in *Dancing with the Stars*. Remember, when I signed up for that show, I didn't know any more about ballroom dancing than you probably do now. (I was fortunate in that I turned out to have a natural feel for dance.) These are basic steps, yet over a matter of weeks, I advanced them with Karina's help.

"First off, you don't need to rush like Mario did with the show," she says. "In fact, you're not going to become a great dancer just by reading this book. For that, you'll have to take lessons at some point, and the sooner the better, as far as I'm concerned. What you can do, right now, is mimic the main muscle action of these basic steps in a way that will give you a feel for the move while burning calories and sculpting the target muscles. Your dance technique doesn't have to pass muster with the *Dancing with the Stars* judges—not yet, anyway. But when you decide to take it to that level, you'll be ready."

10-MINUTE WORKOUT GIANT SETS FOR SHOULDERS

Use the same weight for all four exercises, but as you fatigue, the weight will feel heavier. The beauty of this workout is that each move places your body in a stronger biomechanical position, so you should be able to handle it.

Sequence	Exercise	Sets	Reps	Rest (seconds)
A1	Bent-over Lateral Raise	2	10	↓
A2	Lateral Raise	2	10	↓
A3	Upright Row	2	10	↓
A4	Overhead Press	2	10	60

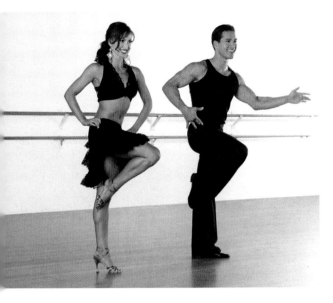

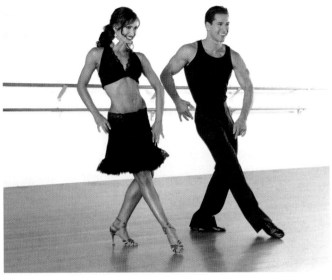

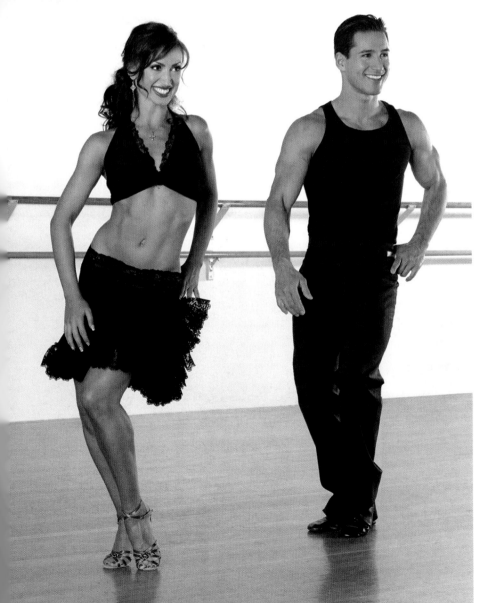

KICK BALL CHANGE IN JIVE

I recommend this step for improved stamina—not to mention firming up your buttocks, thighs, and calves.

This move involves a small kick, so I want you to mimic it with a series of hip extensions. Stand straight with your hands on your hips, and slowly raise your left leg back behind you. Repeat 10 times before switching legs for the same number of reps.

CHACHA BASIC IN PLACE

This is great for developing core muscles and toning up the back.

The chacha is basically a series of steps, and the best way to prepare for it is to do a sequence of lunges. Stand upright with your hands on your hips, and then step to the left.

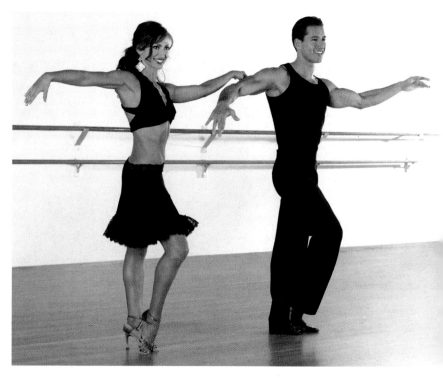

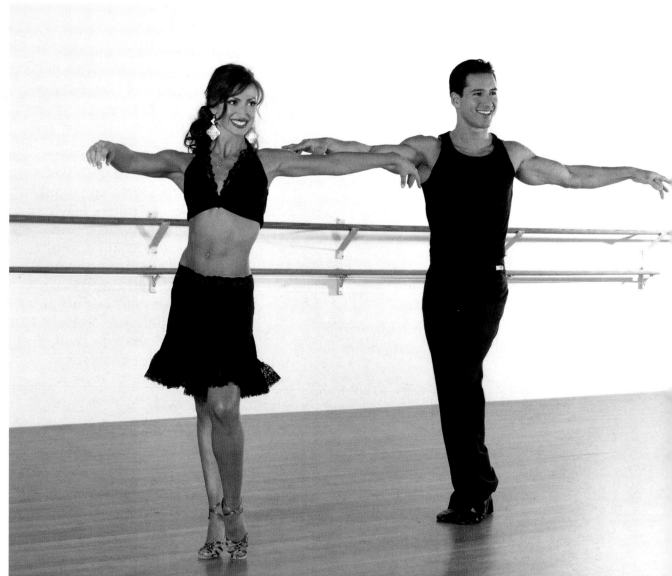

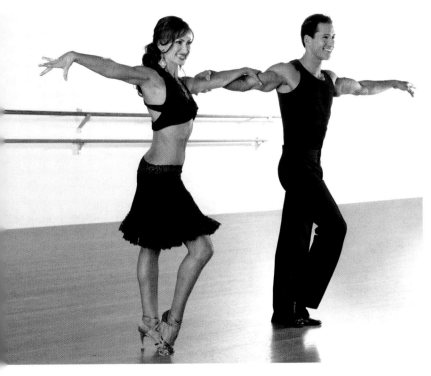

Return to the starting position, and then step forward. Return to the starting position, and then step to the right. This equals 1 repetition, so complete the sequence 9 times, for 10 reps total.

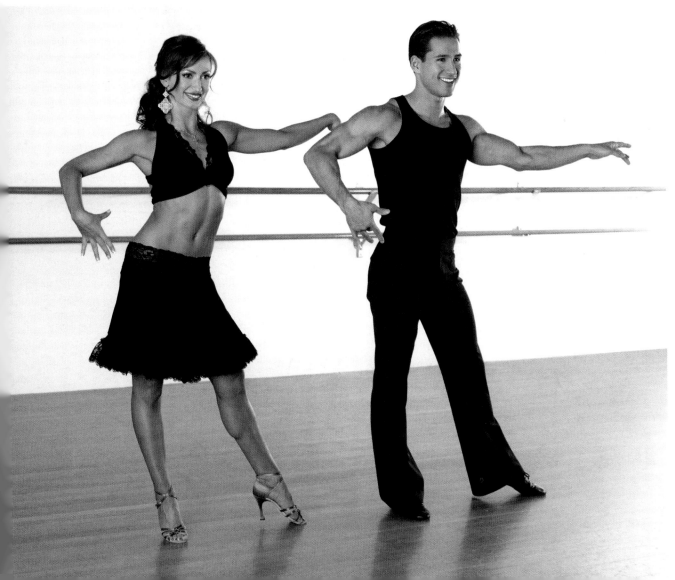

TANGO SWIVELS

This dance makes for a complete upper-body workout, calling on your arms, shoulders, and back. It also works on balance and stability.

To mimic the swiveling motion of this dance step, do V-up twists. Lie on the floor and then raise your legs and torso off the ground, so that your body looks like a V from the side. Curl your torso up and to the right 10 times, using quick rotations. Repeat 10 times before switching sides for the same number of reps to the left.

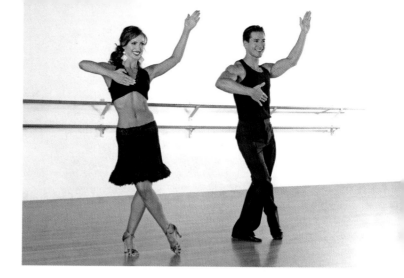

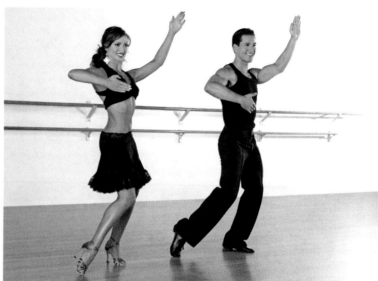

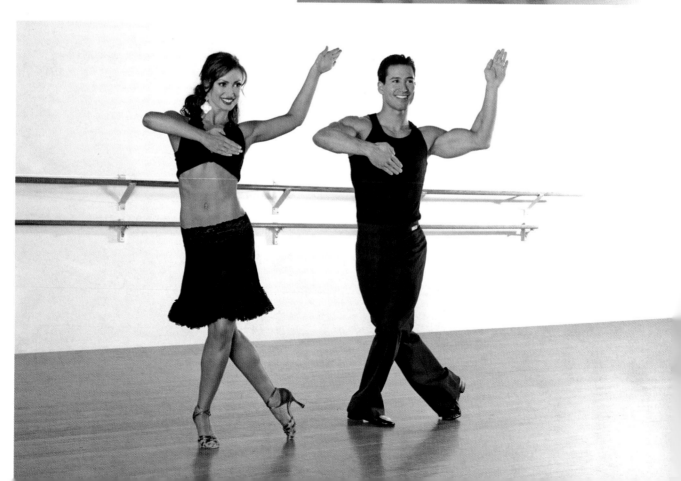

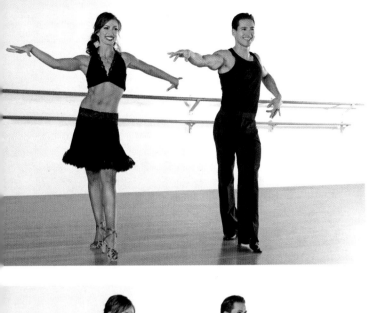

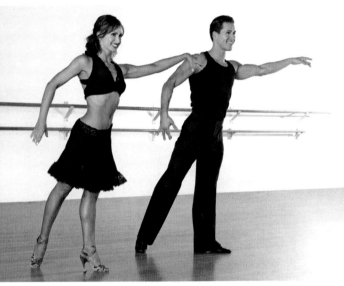

RUMBA CUBAN BREAKS

If you want the kind of ripped midsection showcased on *Dancing with the Stars*, try this. The rotational stretch in your midsection is amazing. Rumba Cuban Breaks also work the back, arms, and legs.

To mimic that rotational twist, lie faceup on an exercise ball with your knees bent 90 degrees and your feet planted on the floor. Raise your arms above you and clasp your hands. Rotate your torso to the right, until your arms are parallel with the floor. Raise your arms back to the center, and then lower your arms to the other side. Continue in this windmill fashion until you've gone back and forth 20 times.

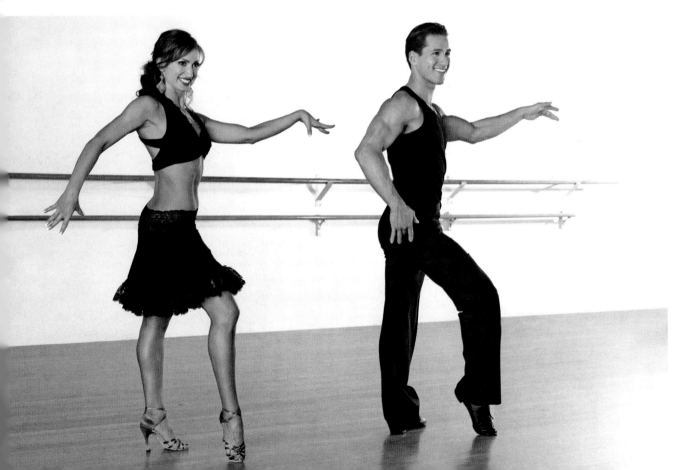

MAMBO SPOT TURNS

These turns to the left and right are great for posture, balance, and complete midsection development.

To prepare you for those 360 turns, I want you to work on rotating your torso from a standing position. Stand on one leg with the other leg raised to the front, and swivel your torso from side to side 20 times. Switch leg positions and do the same number of twists.

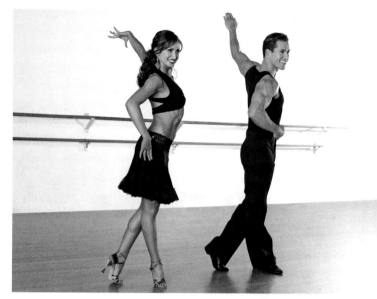

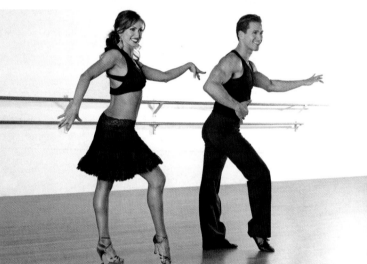

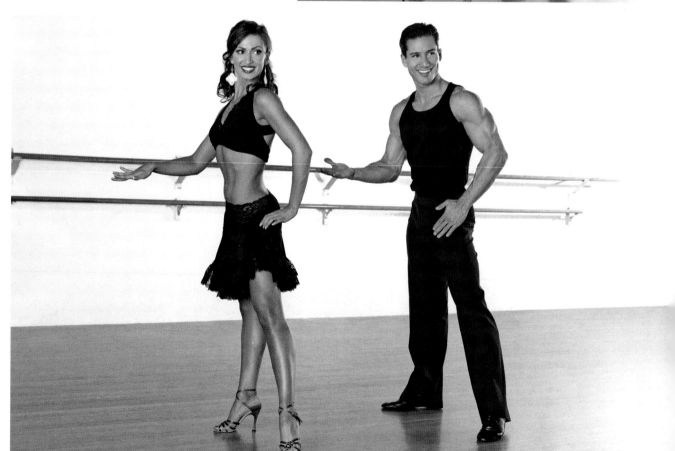

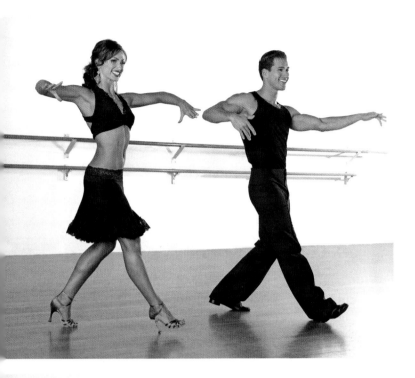

WALTZ BOX STEP

This move is very simple, but it simultaneously works back, legs, and posture. It also develops overall body control and toning.

To prepare for this dance move, stack several aerobic steps in front of you. Step onto the platform with your left foot, and then bring your right foot up behind it. Step back with your left foot followed by your right. Repeat 9 times, and then do the same number of reps leading with your right leg.

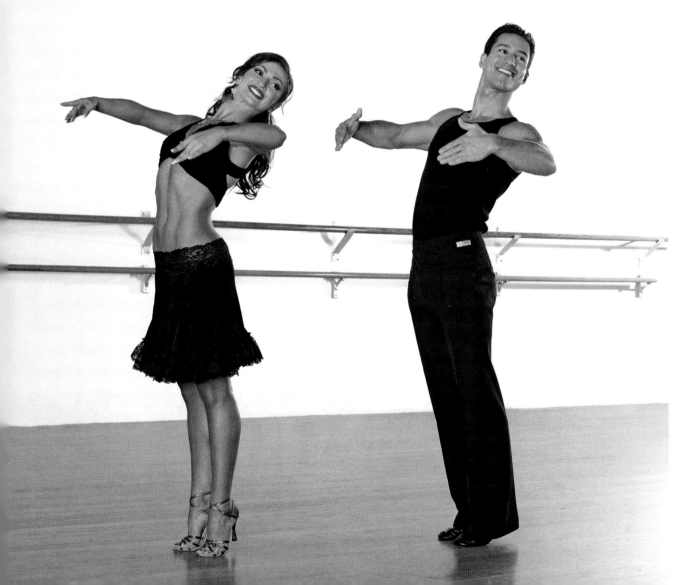

Phase III:
Workout F
MAKING A BIG SPLASH:
MY WATER WORKOUT

I love to swim, too, but I'll be the first to admit that it's not my strongest suit—not yet, anyway. I've participated in some fun marathons, but the only reason I haven't done a triathlon yet is that my swimming needs an upgrade. I was a little leery of swimming for so long, but that's definitely next on the to-do list.

Weights can add power to your swimming stroke. "It's important to be strong through certain joints and ranges of motion to enable swimmers to hold their stroke length for longer," Julian Jones, head of the strength and conditioning department at the Australian Institute of Sport in Canberra, Australia, tells me. At the same time, you don't want to become too beefy, or you won't exactly be knifing through the water. "As your surface area starts to get bigger, it will exponentially increase your drag in the water," Jones says.

When you hop out of the pool and head back to the gym, you'll find that the benefits go the other way. The cardiovascular benefits of swimming aren't to be underestimated. Like running, swimming raises your heart rate, and keeps it elevated throughout the workout. An added bonus from swimming is that you can increase your strength and muscle size at the same time you're burning all those calories. Workouts on dry land simply don't mimic the full-body muscle recruitment that happens in H_2O.

In Phase III, I'm giving you the option of doing a session of cardio-oriented pool work to replace one of the interval sessions that would normally follow weights. Here are several options. Mix and match as your endurance allows:

- Tread water for 1 to 3 minutes in the deep end. Repeat several times.
- Sprint the width of the pool and then walk back to the other side. Repeat several times.
- Swim a lap using your upper body only while squeezing a floatation device, such as a kickboard, between your legs. Swim a lap using your lower body only while holding the same floatation device at arm's length in front of your head. Continue alternating laps.

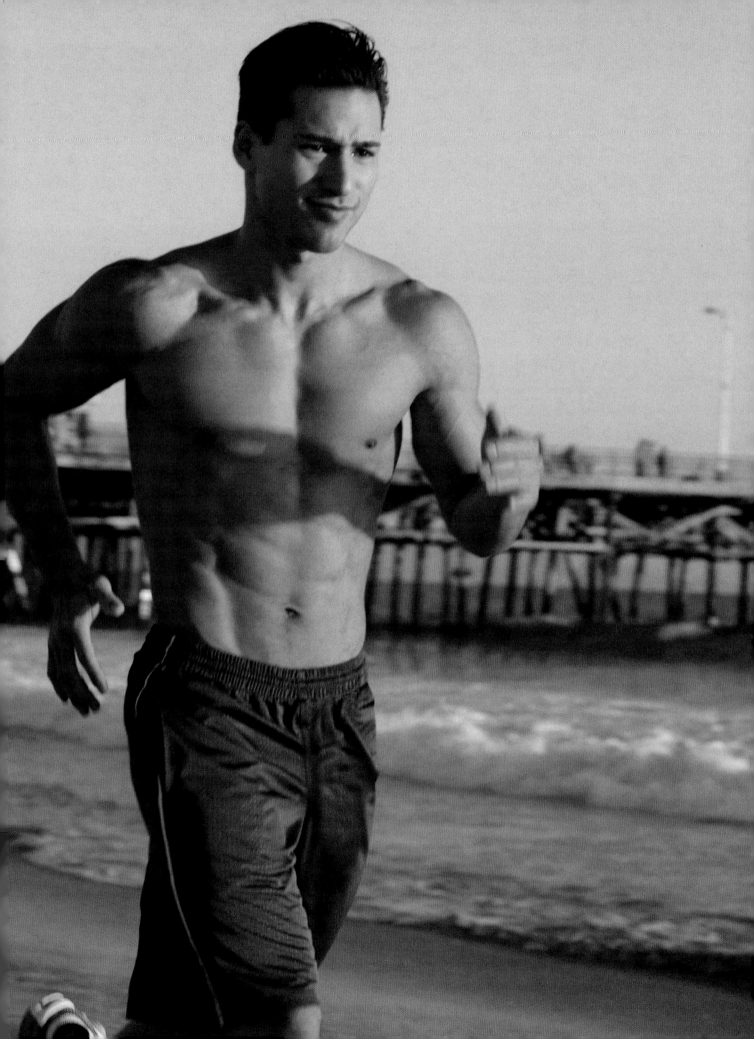

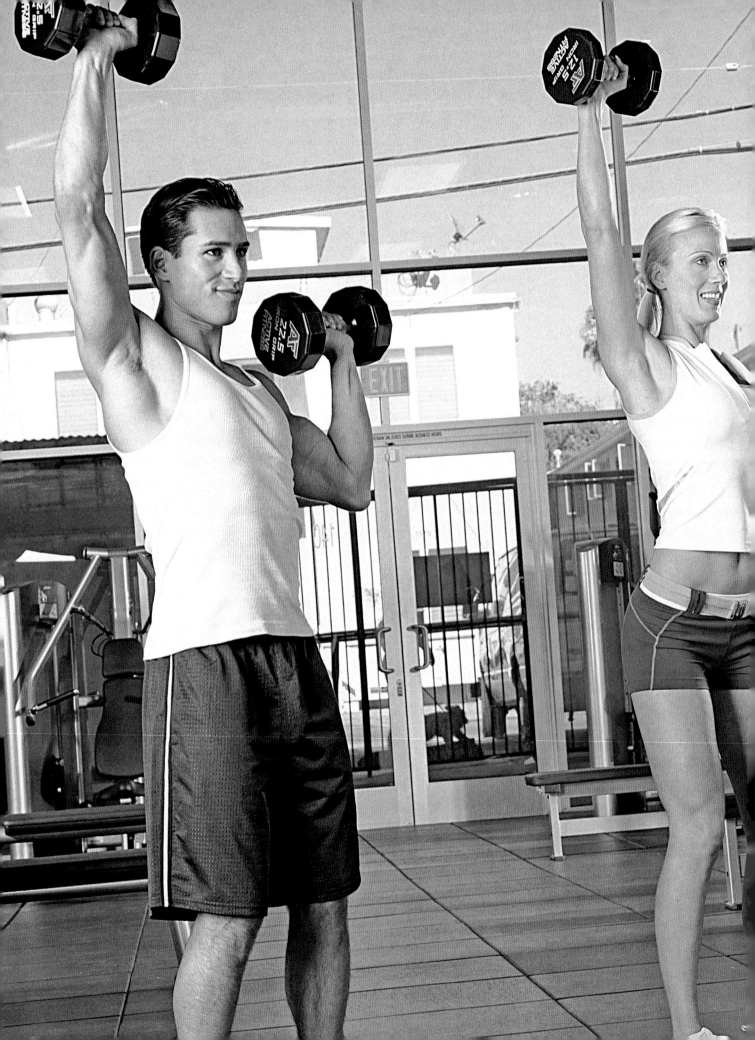

9 Meal Plans

Everyone knows from early childhood that a relationship exists between strength and nutrition—probably when they first see Popeye rip the lid off a can of spinach.

Training for strength and power doesn't require pounding down a ton of carbs like powerlifters and strongmen do. Just look at their physiques, and you can tell that all those carbs aren't burned for energy; instead, many are converted to blubber. The huge spare tires on display at a World's Strongest Man competition aren't limited to the ones being pushed end over end around the competition venue. For you, the end result will be different largely because of what and how much you'll be eating.

The carb allocation during this phase will provide enough fuel for workout recovery, while allowing you to ward off new body fat—and burn some more for good measure. Protein stays the same during Phase III, allowing your muscles to gain more strength and power from the new training tools at your disposal. Fat falls to less than 0.5 gram per pound of body weight, which will help keep a lid on your calorie intake. You can do this by eating like the Phase I nutrition plan for most of the day, but then really clamping down on carbs at dinner and with your nighttime snack. Also, don't forget you can continue to mix and match your sample daily menu meal choices. You will also continue to have the option to chose from a variety of fast food meals that are interchangeable with each other.

The numbers for Phase III are as follows:

- Anywhere from 10 to 12 calories per pound of body weight
- Between 0.5 and 1 gram of carbs per pound of body weight
- Approximately 1 gram of protein per pound of body weight
- Less than 0.5 grams of fat per pound of body weight

10–12 calories × (your weight) = calories per day
0.5–1 gram of carbs × (your weight) = carbohydrates per day
1 gram of protein × (your weight) = protein per day
0.5 gram of fat × (your weight) = fat per day

5 SAUCES YOU SHOULD AVOID AT ALL COSTS

1) Alfredo sauce: ½ cup packs in at least 22 grams of fat, about half of them saturated. *Healthier alternative:* low-fat Alfredo. Add two cups of plain soymilk (the thicker consistency mimics Alfredo) to a pot over low heat. Stir regularly to prevent sticking. Don't bring milk to a boil. Add 1 tablespoon of dry milk powder, ½ cup of grated Parmesan cheese, salt, and pepper to mixture. Continue to stir until cheese is melted and milk is thickened. If mixture is not of the desired consistency, add dry milk powder and stir until dissolved. You'll slash the fat calories by more than half!

2) Full-fat salad dressing: It's loaded with calories and fat. *Healthier alternative:* canned vegetable stock. Place in a pot on the stove and bring to a boil. Mix 1 tablespoon of cornstarch with ¼ cup of cold water until dissolved. Add this mixture to the boiling liquid. This will thicken the stock and create the same consistency as high-fat, oil-based dressings. Then whisk in 1 clove of chopped garlic, 1 tablespoon of oregano, 1 teaspoon of basil, and ¼ cup balsamic vinegar.

3) Hollandaise sauce: This rich sauce is a mixture of eggs, butter, and several other ingredients that all add up on the scale. *Healthier alternative:* Add 4 ounces of firm tofu, 4 teaspoons of lemon juice, a pinch of salt and pepper, one tablespoon of capers, and three tablespoons of canned vegetable stock to a food processor or blender. Blend until smooth and serve.

4) Bolognese sauce: This fatty meat sauce packs a hefty dose of sausage, ground beef—and loads of artery-clogging fat. *Healthier alternative:* Heat 1 tablespoon of olive oil in a pot over medium heat. Chop 1 clove of garlic and ½ red onion. Add to the oil and stir constantly to prevent burning. After about five minutes, add 2 16-ounce cans of crushed tomatoes and the same amount of canned whole tomatoes. Stir. Add 1 tablespoon each of tomato paste, dried oregano, and dried basil. Salt and pepper to taste. Cook over low-medium heat for about 30 to 45 minutes.

5) Gravy: While turkey itself is fantastic for you, smothering it with gravy creates a gut bomb. *Healthier alternative:* Buy two cans of fat-free turkey stock, add to a pot, and bring to a boil. Mix 1 teaspoon of cornstarch with about ¼ cup of water. Add this mixture to the boiling stock to thicken, and remove from heat. Salt and pepper to taste. You lose nearly all the calories and fat, yet keep 100 percent of the flavor.

On days when you work out, here's what your body needs:

- About 14 calories per pound of body weight
- Up to 1 gram of carbs per pound of body weight
- A little more than 1 gram of protein per pound of body weight
- About 0.5 gram of fat per pound of body weight. Feel free to go a little lower.

This can be achieved simply by adding one snack to your diet from our "Workout Eats" section. Consume it immediately after training, if possible.

14 calories × (your weight) = calories per day
1 gram of carbs × (your weight) = carbohydrates per day
>1 gram of protein × (your weight) = protein per day
0.5 gram of fat × (your weight) = fat per day

The following sample meal plans represent what I typically eat. If you weigh less than 175 pounds, reduce your intake. One way is to cut out one of the three daily snacks. For example, if you don't feel hungry between breakfast and lunch, skip the late-morning snack. Alternatively, reduce your intake by reducing the serving sizes for some meals. To cut back on protein, eat two eggs instead of four at breakfast; less deli meat than what's listed here; ½ cup of cottage cheese instead of 1 cup; or a smaller portion of protein (chicken, turkey, seafood, steak) at dinner. To cut back on your carbohydrate intake, eat ⅛ Boboli whole-wheat pizza crust instead of ¼; half a bagel, English muffin, or bran muffin instead of a whole one; half a pita instead of a whole one; and ½ cup of cereal instead of 1 cup.

HEY, MARIO!

I've heard for years that eggs are okay for me, but only if I remove the yolks, because they contain cholesterol. Is this true?

Eggs are a nearly perfect food, yolk included. In fact, a recent study from the University of Connecticut found that adding *extra* yolk to a diet didn't raise bad cholesterol. In another study, subjects having eggs for breakfast ate less food throughout the day than those given a higher-carbohydrate breakfast.

Workout Eats

On training days, consume one of these snacks within 1 hour of the end of your workout.

Food	Calories	Protein (g)	Carbs (g)	Fat (g)
Power Bar Protein Plus	270	22	30	9
Clif Builder	270	20	30	8
16 oz Jamba Juice Protein Berry Workout w/ soy protein	280	14	56	1
16 oz low-fat chocolate milk	316	16	52	4
8 oz plain non-fat yogurt + 1 cup blueberries	210	14	38	0

Sample Daily Meal Plans: Phase III
Monday

Breakfast
2 whole eggs

2 egg whites

Scramble or fry eggs.

1 whole-grain waffle

1 cup sliced strawberries

1 tablespoon fat-free sour cream

1 teaspoon brown sugar

Mix brown sugar into sour cream. Add strawberries to waffle and top with sour cream mixture.

Late-morning snack
1 cup cottage cheese

½ cup sliced pineapple

Mix pineapple into cottage cheese; eat by scooping crackers into mixture.

Lunch
6-inch Subway Turkey and ham (double meat) on wheat with mustard and your choice of vegetables

Mid-afternoon snack
1 cup plain low-fat yogurt

½ cup blueberries

Dinner
9 ounces tilapia (broiled or grilled)

10 asparagus spears

2 cups mixed green salad

2 tablespoons olive oil and vinegar dressing

1 Edy's/Dreyer's Frozen Fruit Bar (strawberry, tangerine, raspberry)

Late-night snack
5-ounce packet Starkist seasoned tuna filets

Heat in microwave if desired.

Totals: 1,748 calories, 151 grams of carbohydrates, 194 grams of protein, 44 grams of fat.

✳ If you work out today, choose one snack from "Workout Eats," and consume within one hour of working out. Be sure to consider these nutritional values when planning your nutrition totals for the day.

Tuesday

Breakfast

Breakfast Pizza

1 whole egg

$\frac{1}{2}$ cup fat-free mozzarella

$\frac{1}{4}$ Boboli whole-wheat pizza crust

2 slices Jennie-O extra lean turkey bacon
(chopped into 1-inch pieces)

Beat egg in bowl and slowly drizzle half over the crust. Spread cheese over crust and drizzle the rest of the egg over the cheese. Top with bacon. Bake in oven at 450°F for about 10 minutes.

Late-morning snack

10 Washboard Waffles*

$\frac{1}{4}$ cup Vermont sugar-free maple syrup

8 ounces skim milk

  * can be ordered at washboardwaffles.com

Lunch

4 ounces lean ground beef (95% lean)

10-inch whole-wheat tortilla

$\frac{1}{4}$ cup fat-free cheddar cheese (optional)

1 tablespoon fat-free sour cream (optional)

2 tablespoons salsa (optional)

Lettuce and tomato

Brown beef. Warm tortilla in pan. Add beef to tortilla. If desired, top with cheese, sour cream, salsa, lettuce and tomato.

Mid-afternoon snack

$\frac{1}{2}$ can white tuna

$\frac{1}{2}$ cup low-fat cottage cheese

Mix tuna into cottage cheese.

Dinner

Shrimp Scampi

1 tablespoon olive oil

1 clove garlic, crushed

1 teaspoon parsley

Lemon juice

$\frac{1}{4}$ cup white cooking wine

Salt and pepper, to taste

6 ounces shrimp

Heat olive oil in skillet. Add garlic, parsley, a dash of lemon juice, wine, and salt and pepper. Bring to a boil, lower heat, and simmer for 3 minutes. Add shrimp and cook, stirring frequently, for 5 to 6 minutes until shrimp is pink. Remove from heat, place on plate, and pour sauce from skillet over shrimp.

2 cups mixed green salad

2 tablespoons olive oil-and-vinegar salad dressing

½ cup blueberries

2 tablespoons fat-free Reddi Wip

Top blueberries with Reddi Wip.

Late-night snack

1 cup cottage cheese

2 tablespoons salsa

Top cottage cheese with salsa.

Totals: 2,059 calories, 114 grams of carbohydrates, 161 grams of protein, 54 grams of fat.

* If you work out today, choose one snack from "Workout Eats," and consume within one hour of working out. Be sure to consider these nutritional values when planning your nutrition totals for the day.

HEY, MARIO!

I get it that water's healthy for me, but can it help me lose weight?

Yes. People who drink more water tend to eat less, but the weight-loss benefit goes beyond that. Dehydration slows metabolism. In one study, subjects who drank two cups of water had a resting metabolic rate more than 30 percent higher than those who didn't. The effect lasted for nearly two hours.

Wednesday

Breakfast

1 cup Kashi GoLean Cereal

1 cup skim milk

Late-morning snack

2 sticks light mozzarella string cheese (2 ounces)

1 ounce mixed nuts

Lunch

McDonald's Premium Grilled Chicken Classic (without mayo)

Late-afternoon snack

5 ounces canned lump crabmeat

1 tablespoon light mayonnaise

2 or 3 large celery stalks

Mix mayo into crabmeat and spoon into the groove of the celery.

Dinner

6 ounces top sirloin steak (grilled or broiled)

½ cup canned mushrooms (sautéed in olive oil)

10 asparagus spears

2 cups mixed green salad

2 tablespoons olive oil-and-vinegar salad dressing

8 bittersweet (60% cacao) chocolate chips

1 tablespoons peanut butter

Late-night snack

Deviled Eggs

2 whole eggs

2 egg whites

1 tablespoon light mayonnaise

Dill or tarragon (optional)

Hard-boil eggs. Slice eggs lengthwise. Remove yolks and discard two. Mix remaining yolks with mayo and herbs if desired and spoon mix back into the eight egg-white halves.

Totals: 1,944 calories, 134 grams of carbohydrates, 168 grams of protein, 87 grams of fat.

* If you work out today, choose one snack from "Workout Eats," and consume within one hour of working out. Be sure to consider these nutritional values when planning your nutrition totals for the day.

Thursday

Breakfast

1 whole-wheat English muffin

2 slices low-fat deli ham

2 whole eggs

1 slice low-fat American cheese

Toast muffin. Fry ham in pan and place on one half of muffin. Fry eggs in pan using non-fat cooking spray and place on ham. Top eggs with cheese and cover with other muffin half to make breakfast sandwich.

Late-morning snack

1 tablespoon peanut butter

1 tablespoon light cream cheese

2 to 3 large celery stalks

Mix peanut butter and cream cheese. Spoon into the grove of the celery.

$\frac{1}{2}$ large grapefruit

Lunch

Turkey Sandwich

4 ounces deli turkey

1 tablespoon light mayonnaise (or mustard if preferred)

2 slices whole-wheat bread

Late-afternoon snack

Deli Roll-ups

2 slices low-fat American cheese

4 slices low-fat deli ham, turkey, or roast beef

Lay 1 slice of cheese in between 2 slices of ham. Roll up.

$\frac{1}{2}$ large grapefruit

Dinner

1 spaghetti squash (to yield 1 cup)

6 ounces lean ground beef (95% lean)

$\frac{1}{4}$ cup spaghetti/marinara sauce

Cut spaghetti squash in half lengthwise. Place halves in microwave and cook on high 6 to 8 minutes. Let cool, then scrape out flesh with fork to make spaghetti. Brown meat and add on top of squash. Top with sauce.

$\frac{1}{2}$ cup sliced strawberries

2 tablespoons fat-free Reddi Wip

Top strawberries with Reddi Wip.

Late-night snack

Skillet Tuna Melt

3 ounces white tuna

1 tablespoon light mayonnaise

$\frac{1}{2}$ cup fat-free cheddar cheese

Mix tuna with mayo. Spray heated skillet with nonfat cooking spray. Sprinkle $\frac{1}{4}$ cup shredded cheese on skillet. Spread tuna over cheese and let cook until cheese is golden brown around edges. Remove from pan.

Sprinkle remaining cheese on skillet and add tuna, top side down. Let cook until cheese is golden brown around edges.

1 ounce mixed nuts

Totals: 1,959 calories, 134 grams of carbohydrates, 183 grams of protein, 78 grams of fat.

* If you work out today, choose one snack from "Workout Eats," and consume within one hour of working out. Be sure to consider these nutritional values when planning your nutrition totals for the day.

Friday

Breakfast
Western Bagel Perfect 10 Healthy Grain Bagel
1 tablespoon peanut butter

Late morning snack
1 cup cottage cheese
½ cup sliced pineapple
Mix pineapple into cottage cheese and eat by scooping crackers into mixture.

Lunch
6-inch Subway Roast Beef (double meat) on wheat, with mustard and your choice of any Subway vegetables as toppings.

Mid-afternoon snack
3 ounces canned chicken breast
1 tablespoon light mayonnaise
9 whole-wheat crackers
Mix mayo into chicken and eat on crackers.

Dinner
9 ounces salmon (broiled or grilled)
1 cup mixed vegetables (canned or frozen), prepared

2 ounces dark chocolate (60%+ cacao)
1 teaspoon peanut butter

Late-night snack
Asparagus Roll-ups
1 tablespoon light cream cheese
4 slices low-fat deli ham
4 asparagus spears
Spread cream cheese onto ham. Place asparagus onto ham and roll up. Repeat with other 3 slices.

Totals: 2,042 calories, 146 grams of carbohydrates, 186 grams of protein, 79 grams of fat.

* If you work out today, choose one snack from "Workout Eats," and consume within one hour of working out. Be sure to consider these nutritional values when planning your nutrition totals for the day.

Saturday

Breakfast

Cheesy Crab Omelet

2 whole eggs plus 1 egg white, beaten

¼ cup fat-free mozzarella

5 ounces canned lump crabmeat

Spray pan with nonfat cooking spray. Heat to medium and pour in eggs. Cook eggs till set and flip. Add cheese and crab. Fold egg over to make omelet.

1 low-fat bran muffin

Late-morning snack

1 cup plain low-fat yogurt

¼ cup granola

Lunch

3 ounces white tuna

1 tablespoon light mayonnaise

1 large wheat pita bread

Pickle relish and chopped vegetables (optional)

Mix tuna with mayo. If desired, add relish and vegetables. Spread into pita bread.

Mid-afternoon snack

Deli Roll-ups

1 ounce fat-free cheese (Swiss, cheddar, or Monterey jack)

2 slices deli turkey, ham, or roast beef

Slice cheese into 2 thin pieces and place in middle of turkey. Roll up.

1 ounce mixed nuts

Dinner

Bacon Cheeseburger Quiche

1 pound lean ground beef

1 small onion, chopped

4 slices extra-lean turkey bacon

4 eggs

8 tablespoons reduced-fat sour cream

½ cup fat-free half-and-half

1 cup shredded fat-free cheddar cheese

1 teaspoon garlic powder

Preheat oven to 350°F. In skillet over medium heat, brown beef with onion, and remove from pan. Cook bacon in skillet and cut into 1-inch pieces. Add beef and bacon to bottom of a pie pan. Combine eggs, sour cream, half-and-half, cheese, and garlic powder in bowl and mix well. Pour mixture over beef "crust" and bake 40 to 45 minutes, until top is browned. *Makes four servings.*

½ cup sliced strawberries

2 tablespoons fat-free Reddi Wip

Top strawberries with Reddi Wip.

Late-night snack

Skillet Tuna Melt

3 ounces white tuna

1 tablespoon light mayonnaise

½ cup fat-free cheddar cheese

Mix tuna with mayo. Spray heated skillet with nonfat cooking spray. Sprinkle ¼ cup shredded cheese on skillet. Spread tuna over cheese and let cook until cheese is golden brown around edges. Remove from pan. Sprinkle remaining cheese on skillet and add tuna, top side down. Let cook until cheese is golden brown around edges.

    1 ounce mixed nuts

Totals: 2,113 calories, 134 grams of carbohydrates, 207 grams of protein, 85 grams of fat.

✱ If you work out today, choose one snack from "Workout Eats," and consume within one hour of working out. Be sure to consider these nutritional values when planning your nutrition totals for the day.

Sunday

Breakfast
    2 whole eggs (fried, scrambled, or hard boiled)
    1 Washboard Waffle*
    ¼ cup Vermont sugar-free maple syrup
        * can be ordered at washboardwaffles.com

Late-morning snack
    5 ounces can lump crabmeat
    1 tablespoon light mayonnaise
    2 to 3 large celery stalks
    Mix mayo into crabmeat and spoon into the groove of the celery.

Lunch
    Wendy's Black Forest Ham and Swiss Frescata (no cheese)

Mid-afternoon snack
    1 stick light mozzarella string cheese (1 ounce)
    2 ounces beef jerky

Dinner
    Chicken Stir-fry
    1 cup frozen stir-fry vegetables
    6 ounces chicken breast, sliced
    1 tablespoon soy sauce
    Spray nonfat cooking spray in skillet and add vegetables. Cook over medium heat, stirring occasionally until vegetables have begun to thaw (about 5 minutes). Add chicken and soy sauce and continue cooking until chicken is cooked through.

    2 cups mixed green salad
    2 tablespoons olive oil-and-vinegar dressing

    ½ cup blueberries
    2 tablespoons fat-free Reddi Wip
    Top blueberries with Reddi Wip.

Late-night snack
    1 cup cottage cheese
    2 tablespoons salsa
    Top cottage cheese with salsa.

Totals: 1,671 calories, 119 grams of carbohydrates, 175 grams of protein, 50 grams of fat.

✱ If you work out today, choose one snack from "Workout Eats," and consume within one hour of working out. Be sure to consider these nutritional values when planning your nutrition totals for the day.

QUICK & TASTY MEALS

Breakfast

Spanish Breakfast Scramble

Nonfat cooking spray
1/4 chopped tomato
1/4 cup chopped green pepper
1/4 cup chopped onion
1 whole egg
1/2 cup egg substitute
1/4 cup fat-free shredded cheddar cheese
1 tablespoon hot sauce

Coat a large nonstick skillet with cooking spray; place over medium-high heat until hot. Add tomato, green pepper, and onions; sauté until tender, stirring occasionally. Remove mixture from skillet and set aside.

Combine egg, egg substitute, cheese, and hot sauce in a large bowl; beat well with a wire whisk. Pour mixture into skillet and cook over low heat, stirring gently. Cook until eggs are firm but still moist. Remove from heat. Stir in vegetable mixture. Transfer to plate and enjoy.

Makes one serving.

Add 1 slice of whole wheat bread with 1 tablespoon lite trans-fat-free margarine; 1/2 red grapefruit and 1 meatless sausage heated in the microwave.

Total: 532 calories; 40 grams protein, 48 grams carbohydrates, 22 grams fat (29% protein, 35% carbohydrates, 36% fat)

Lunch & Dinner
500 Calories

Grilled Ginger Lamb Chops

8 4-ounce lean lamb loin chops, trimmed of fat
1/2 cup Burgundy or other dry red wine
2 tablespoons peeled, minced ginger
1 tablespoon low-sodium soy sauce
1 tablespoon honey
1 teaspoon onion powder
1/4 teaspoon pepper
1 clove garlic
Nonfat cooking spray
1 teaspoon cornstarch
1/4 cup canned no-salt added beef broth, undiluted and divided

Place chops in a shallow dish. Combine wine, ginger, soy sauce, honey, onion powder, pepper, and garlic in a bowl; stir well. Pour wine mixture over chops. Cover and marinate in refrigerator at least 8 hours; turn occasionally. Remove chops from marinade, straining and reserving 1/2 cup marinade. Coat grill rack with cooking spray; place on grill over medium-hot coals.

Place chops on rack and cook 8 to 10 minutes on each side or to desired degree of doneness. Transfer chops to a serving platter and keep warm. Dissolve cornstarch in 1 Tbsp. beef broth; add remaining 3 Tbsp. broth; stir well. Combine ½ cup reserved marinade and beef broth mixture in a small saucepan, stirring well. Cook over medium heat, stirring constantly, until mixture comes to a boil. Cook 1 minute or until broth is thickened, stirring constantly. Pour broth mixture evenly over chops.

Makes four servings.

Add 2 cups tossed salad with balsamic vinegar; whole-wheat dinner roll (1 ounce); 1 tablespoon butter; 1 orange; water or Crystal Light

Total: 504 calories; 34 grams protein, 47 grams carbohydrates, 20 grams fat (27% protein, 37% carbohydrates, 36% fat)

Dijon-Glazed Chicken

  2 tablespoons Dijon mustard
  1 tablespoon brown sugar
  1 tablespoon honey
  1 teaspoon minced ginger
  4 4-ounce chicken cutlets
  Nonfat cooking spray

Combine mustard, brown sugar, honey and ginger in a small bowl; stir well. Coat grill rack with cooking spray; place on grill over medium-hot coals. Place chicken on rack, brushing half of glaze mixture over chicken. Cook 5 minutes; turn chicken and brush with remaining glaze. Cook an additional 5 minutes or until chicken is cooked through.

Makes 4 servings.

Add 3 cups tossed salad; 2 tablespoons lite Ranch salad dressing; 5 ounces corn on the cob (boiled); ½ cup unsweetened applesauce; water or Crystal Light

Total: 509 calories; 37 grams protein, 72 grams carbohydrates, 8 grams fat (29% protein, 57% carbohydrates; 14% fat)

Snack
Peanut Butter & Jelly Sandwich

  1 slice whole-wheat bread
  1 tablespoon peanut butter
  1 teaspoon jelly

172 calories; 6 grams protein, 19 grams carbohydrates, 9 grams fat (14% protein, 41% carbohydrates, 45% fat)

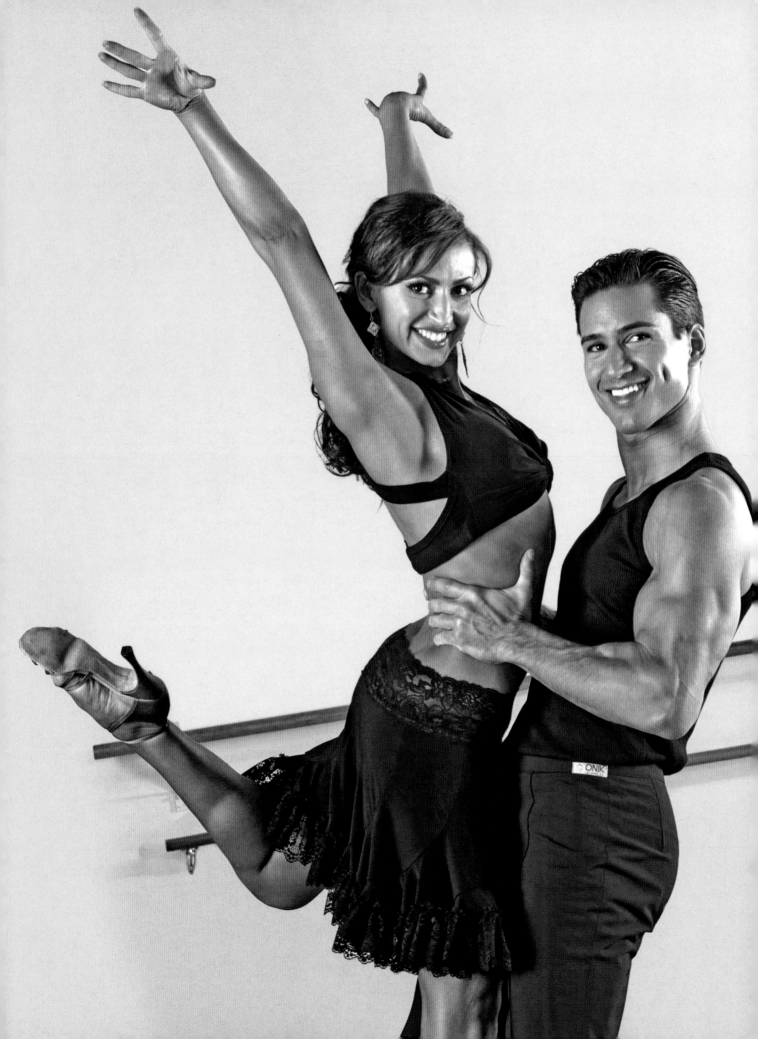

10 Now It's Up to You

Imitating the workout protocols of actors and other entertainers was once a dubious proposition at best. Errol Flynn was so hung over at his workouts that his trainer would bring him a bottle of mouthwash. (He would slug that down, too.) As recently as the 1970s, six packs were something superstars drank, not beach-ready abs.

Today, so many of us actors, musicians, and athletes—all rightly called entertainers—hoist barbells instead of beer mugs because millions of dollars ride on how we look and perform. In fact, shaping up for a movie, a video shoot, or a season of a program is as essential as reading the script, rehearsing the song, or memorizing the playbook. That's why I've taken that job requirement and adopted it as my lifestyle.

By completing this workout and nutrition program—either the 6- or 12-week version—you too have taken a bold step toward taking control of your body, not to mention your life. You started with a goal, self-improvement; and armed yourself with a plan, this book. When goals and a plan for achieving them come together; and are brought to life by discipline, determination, and action; it's a beautiful thing.

What now? My hunch is that I don't need to answer that question for you. The improvements you see in the mirror, the increases in your energy levels, the respect you're receiving from friends and family— that's all the motivation you'll be likely to need to keep going. As far as your workouts go, you're running the show now. You can map your own route moving forward. The destination is yours to name.

Here are just a few of your limitless possibilities:

- Consider repeating the program. See how much your weights have increased since you began it the first time. You might be shocked at how much strength you have gained.
- Consider hiring a certified personal trainer, someone who can continue challenging and teaching you. For as much as I now know about training, I still learn something new from my trainer, Jimmy Peña, every time he and I bust a workout.
- Consider buying another fitness book and following that workout program, assuming it looks sound and the sources of information seem reputable. Subscribing to health magazines can offer you great new workouts every month.
- You might begin stocking a home gym, if that fits your lifestyle better than joining a gym and hiring a trainer. You'll be amazed at what you can achieve with a good set of dumbbells, an adjustable bench, and the desire to transform your body.

The specific path you choose is less important than choosing some path and following it to see where it takes you. Keep moving. Stay the course. Don't stop. Never stagnate. Integrate your training into your lifestyle by making it a habit. One theme of this book, always worth remembering, is that your training needs to go through different phases, or your body will grow accustomed to the same thing. Your body is smarter than your head thinks it is. In many ways, it's the perfect machine. Apply the proper stimuli—exercise, diet, and sleep—and your body will keep changing, improving, repairing itself, and adapting for as long as you want it to. You really won't know what your body is capable of until you provide the raw materials it needs to do its thing like Nature intended.

Train for strength for a while, then train for cuts, then train for muscle. Make sports the cornerstone for a while, and then reduce them to support roles, as

HEY, MARIO!

If I'm fading in the middle of the day, what's the quickest way to boost my energy?

When I'm totally exhausted from my busy schedule, I find that a half-hour nap, say, on a plane ride, works wonders. I'm not alone, either. Greek researchers studied 23,000 individuals over a long period of time and found that those who took three thirty-minute naps per week had a 37 percent lower chance of dying from a heart attack.

they are here. Mix it up, and then change it again. In experiment after experiment, exercise scientists around the world keep showing that varying your workouts produces the best results. Plus, it's more fun that way. What more do you need to know?

Underlying the variety and change, of course, is consistency. Consistency and change are two sides of the same coin; long-term fat loss and muscle building require both. And that consistency needs to apply to workouts and nutrition alike. When I was younger, I thought that lifting heavy weights over and over was all that mattered. Now I know that smart training combined with sound nutrition and adequate recuperation produces the best results. It takes time, but like a good investment, the gains just keep compounding as you nail workout after workout. Next thing you know, you look in the mirror and realize you've accomplished something you never thought possible. But it only happens if working out becomes a habit that you can't shake—that you don't want to shake.

Once the habit forms, you'll learn to make the adjustments that only you can make based on your lifestyle and personal preferences. For me, given my schedule, getting enough sleep is a constant challenge. I know my body so well now that I realize just how hugely important sleep is. I know if I'm not resting enough, and if I'm not, I can feel how I need to back off on my training until I'm caught up on shut-eye. With all the traveling I do, especially when the holidays hit, a lack of sleep can wear me down, and I know how to gauge it. I can tell when I'm coming down with something, when I should be holding back. See, for me, the discipline isn't forcing myself to work out; it's giving myself permission to do an easier session. Before, I used to psych myself up and always try to power through it. Now, I might sit in the steam room for half an hour, or pedal a stationary bike for twenty minutes or so, just so I feel like I've broke a sweat. That'll make me feel a little bit better at least.

Being consistent doesn't mean being complacent. Anything but, in fact. Consistency and

HEY, MARIO!

What's the best number for judging my success on this program—body-fat percentage?

There is no magic number. Such statistics are great, but there's more at stake here. It's really about the journey you've taken and what kind of person you become as a result. You don't want to be one of those (many) people who look great on the outside but are miserable on the inside.

maintenance are exactly what allow people to accomplish the unexpected and the spectacular. Tiger Woods and Kobe Bryant are classic examples. When they do something on the links or court that seems inconceivable, where you do think that feat came from? Behind that magic lies years—probably decades—of practicing the same details over and over again. If you're going to stop whatever you're doing to take time out of your day to work out, you should work out hard, yet wisely and efficiently, to maximize the results from your effort. That's an important part of my philosophy.

As Kobe and Tiger prove, if you're focused, you can accomplish whatever you want. That's why I love helping people. There will be those who pick up this book at the store and think they have no shot at taking their body from out of shape to tiptop shape. In six months of solid training, those people can transform their bodies and their lives. They can go from being flabby or skinny to having nice abs. That internal switch in their heads just needs to be turned on.

Although "nice abs" are often considered a symbol of vanity and narcissism, that's a bunch of BS. What those nice abs symbolize is the profound health benefits that come from working out and eating right. I push myself to the limit in the gym now because I want to expand my effectiveness every day—as well as extend to my lifespan to the limit. I hope the old theory—every minute you work out adds a minute to your life—is true. If that's true, I should live to be about 120! And when that birthday comes, I'll be in good shape, too. Here's why:

- A study published recently in the *Journal of Strength and Conditioning Research* found that a group men in their 70s still experience an average 11 percent bump in their testosterone after pumping iron.
- Another study in the *International Journal of Cancer* revealed that working out once a week—just once a once a week!—reduces your chances of being diagnosed with advanced prostate cancer.
- Researchers at Rush University found that eating just two servings of vegetables a day slows the age-related decline in brain function by 40 percent, compared with those who ate fewer or no vegetables.

Explorers have been searching for the fountain of youth since the beginning of recorded history. As it turns out, all Ponce de León had to do was sign up at Gold's Gym!

The study about vegetables and brain function is important because it isn't just about living longer; it's about living *well* longer. The publisher of this book, Rodale, has a corporate slogan that says, "Live Your Whole Life." That sums it up nicely. Survive to 90 or 100, and be vigorous, productive, and happy for that whole long life. I think back to two of my friends and idols, Dick Clark and Merv Griffin, who I wrote about earlier. Merv has now passed, but neither of these guys rested on their laurels as they passed into their 50s, 60s, and 70s. They kept attacking, improving, and reinventing themselves, extending their horizons. That's the kind of grand life one should aspire to live, and working out and eating right can help you in that noble pursuit.

So take your new body and improved mind out into the world with you, and do great things with them. Defy everyone's expectations. Nothing is more rewarding or fun than seeing the expressions on the faces of people when they realize, *You* did *that?* That's a recurring theme in my life, not just in the gym. We've all seen the stories about the child stars on TV who've run into trouble later in life. I was determined not to let that happen to me, but turning out "okay" didn't cut it either. To paraphrase motivational speaker Tony Robbins, I don't want to be good or even excellent. I want to be outstanding or exceptional at everything I do: acting, hosting, and so on down the line.

You can do the same.

Thank you for joining me on this journey. I'll see you at the gym.

Glossary

Active rest: Staying on the move rather than sitting still on days without a regularly scheduled workout. Going for a walk with your significant other is active rest; sitting on the sofa watching me in *Saved by the Bell* reruns is not. If you can't resist the temptation, at least do pushups during commercials.

Aerobic exercise: Any physical activity where exertion prompts the cardio-respiratory system (heart and lungs) to huff and puff as the body demands more oxygen. Remember seeing me fly across the floor on *Dancing with the Stars*? That right there was some serious aerobic exercise, trust me.

Amino acid: Protein constitutes muscle tissue, and amino acids are the building blocks of protein. When it comes to building muscle, think of these as Snow White's dwarves or Santa's reindeer. The array of amino acids found in any given protein largely determines its biological value and activity.

Anabolic: Anything that promotes muscle growth. Typically, a combination of factors (training, protein intake, sleep, etc.) creates what's called an anabolic environment. That's usually a good situation, although the adjective is also applied to illegal agents designed to amplify the growth process. Avoid those at all costs.

Antioxidant: Ever notice how an apple begins turning brown if you take a bite and set it down for a while? That process is called oxidation, and it happens all the time inside the body. Doing the damage are internal molecular scavengers called free radicals. Antioxidants neutralize those rogue agents. The battle is ongoing and continuous.

Barbell: A metal bar with matching plates on either end. If the bar is straight, it's called an Olympic bar; if it's crooked, like those pens chiropractors hand out, it's called an EZ bar. Regardless, the plates can either be removable or welded into a single, indivisible unit.

Body mass index: The mathematical product of your height and weight. According to the Centers for Disease Control and Prevention, BMI, as it's called, "provides a reliable indicator of body fatness for most people and is used to screen for weight categories that may lead to health problems." Well, not really. The government's height-and-weight tables don't account for the ratio of lean mass to body fat, or body composition.

Bodybuilding: Lifting weights to build muscle. Also, the sport in which men and women take muscle building really, really far, in an attempt to become Mr. or Ms. Olympia. The men sometimes compete at 250 to 300 pounds with less than five percent body fat, a conditioning level that typically cannot be achieved without pharmaceutical assistance.

Calisthenics: Body-weight exercises designed to develop muscles as well as promote fitness. These are the moves we would have been asked to do by the gym teacher back at Bayside High School. High-end trainers now charge clients boatloads of cash to have them do jumping jacks and other calisthenics. Drop and give me $200 an hour.

Calorie: This is one of the most widely used words in the English language, but do you know what it means? Most people don't. Technically, a calorie measures the amount of energy needed to raise the temperature of one gram of water by one degree Celsius. One gram of fat contains nine calories; one gram of carbs or protein, four.

Cardiovascular exercise: Using large muscles like the legs to strengthen the heart and lungs—making nearly all "cardio" aerobic as well. Cardiovascular training is an essential element of health, fitness, and wellness. Everybody should do it regularly.

Catabolic: Anything that interferes with or reduces muscle growth; the opposite of anabolic. Too little exercise, too much exercise, a bad diet, insufficient sleep—these and many other factors can lead to catabolism, a state to be avoided.

Cheating: It's not as bad it sounds in a workout context, but it's still not good. Exercise technique varies slightly depending on body type and dimensions, yet every exercise should be performed in an ideal way to produce maximum benefits and prevent injury. Cheating involves compromising that form, usually to lift heavier weights. You can stimulate the muscle better by using less weight but maintaining strict form.

Circuit training: Going from station to station, doing one set of a different exercise at each stop, resting only as long as it takes to move between exercises. Most often done with machines, this is an exhausting technique but well worth the effort, because you're elevating heart rate while simultaneously building muscle.

Compound (a.k.a. multijoint) exercises: These involve movement at more than one set of joints. While performing the barbell row, for example, you're bent at the knees and waist, plus your elbow and shoulder joints help pull the weight. Such moves tend to be more effective than smaller ones at burning calories and stimulating the release of muscle-growth hormones.

Concentric (a.k.a. positive): During this half of the lift, the working muscle contracts, usually working against gravity. Picture the raising of a barbell toward your shoulders.

Core strength: The ability of the midsection muscles—the abdominals, obliques, the spinal erectors of the lower back, and others—to stabilize the body and allow it to perform work. A strong core also means a balanced core, which is why I train my lower back as much as my abs. Functional trainers emphasize developing core strength.

Dietary supplements: From the protein powders you blend to the fish oil pills you pop before bed, supplement makers distill certain beneficial nutrients from food and engineer them into these products. Some of the more esoteric offerings generate controversy, but research over the years has shown many benefits to using multivitamins, etc., to support health.

Dumbbell: You've seen these hunks of iron racked up in front of the mirrors. Dumbbells are smaller than barbells and are usually held with one hand rather than two. The handle and weights typically constitute a single unit, although on occasion dumbbell handles can be fitted with different-sized weight plates. Those are called adjustable DBs.

Eccentric (a.k.a. negative): During this half of the lift, the working muscle lengthens. Picture the lowering of a barbell from your shoulders back down to your waist. (Usually, you're returning to the starting position.) This descent, rather than the lift up, offers the greatest potential for stimulating muscle growth.

Explosiveness: The ability to generate a dramatic increase in power at any time during an exercise or activity.

Fast-twitch muscle fibers: When these contract rapid-fire, they produce great force. Big moves such as the squat and bench press tend to activate them more than smaller moves will. The muscle growth men derive from lifting weights tends to come from fast-twitchers. In contrast, when women train, they develop fast and slow twitch alike.

"Fat burner": These dietary supplements combine stimulants and other ingredients to rev the sympathetic nervous system for short periods of time. Such supplements have been the subject of controversy, and the U.S. FDA pulled the most popular ingredient, ephedra, from the market due to safety concerns.

Free weights: Barbells, dumbbells, kettle bells, etc. As opposed to machines and cable stacks.

Functional training: A training style that focuses on exercising the entire body as an integrated unit, rather than using specific exercises to work distinct muscles. Any time you see someone lifting weights on a wobble board or exercise ball, you know you're in Functional Land. Watch your step.

Glucose: The official name for sugar. One of the goals of my meal plans and exercise programs is to keep too much of this stuff from floating around in your bloodstream.

HDL cholesterol: Some cholesterol is bad, but this is the good stuff. Think of HDL as Liquid-Plumr for your veins, unclogging buildups before they kill your heart.

Hypertension: A $10 word that means high blood pressure, dangerous in its own right, and a warning sign that you're not as healthy as you could be. Along with their other benefits, the workouts and meal plans in this book can all help lower high blood pressure. The interval-training sessions in particular will show hypertension that there's a new sheriff in town.

Insulin: One of the more powerful and complicated hormones in your body, best known for its role in ushering glucose into cells and allowing for its conversion to energy. How effectively insulin works has a genetic component, but how well you steer its action could have a huge bearing on how long and healthfully you live.

Insulin resistance: A condition in which insulin struggles to accomplish its job, because cells don't recognize what it has shown up to do. This prompts the pancreas to produce even more of the hormone, until the pancreas burns out over time. Insulin resistance is a harbinger of significant health problems, most notably adult-onset diabetes. Again, exercise is just what the doctor ordered for this problem.

Integrationists: A term for trainers and athletes who practice functional training.

Intensity: To the layperson, this describes how much effort you expend. When I'm walking down the street, my intensity is low; when I'm in the fifth round of one of my boxing matches, my intensity is friggin' off the charts. In exercise science, though, intensity has a very specific, somewhat different meaning: the load being lifted or otherwise moved, as measured in pounds.

Interval training: Cardiovascular exercise that alternates working really hard with downshifting to a more relaxed pace, or even rest, before the hard portion resumes. Over time, various aspects of an interval program can be altered: the ratio between rest and work; the intensity level of the work portion; or the duration of the entire session.

Isolation exercises (a.k.a. single-joint exercises): These involve movement at only one joint set or set of joints. While performing the barbell curl, for example, your elbows are the only joints that should move during the repetition. Old school trainers like these moves because they allow individual muscles to be worked; functional trainers dismiss these moves for that very reason.

Isolationists: A term for trainers and athletes who practice old school training.

LDL cholesterol: This is the bad cholesterol, the stuff that clogs arteries. LDL cholesterol isn't all the same, though. The smaller and denser the particle circulating in your blood, the more dangerous it becomes.

Lean mass (a.k.a. muscle): The goal is to shift your body composition toward more of this tissue and less body fat. No wonder the word *lean* has graced the covers of a zillion fitness magazines. For most fitness enthusiasts, leaning out is the Holy Grail.

Lecithin: Remember it with this mnemonic device: Its sensitivity to carbohydrate intake, as well as its metabolism-controlling effect, makes this the "thin" hormone.

Machines: Any mechanical contraption that helps you work out, ranging from simple spring-loaded devices to hydraulic machines so complicated and expensive they'd look right at home on the set of a science fiction flick. Machines range from ridiculous to fantastic. Be wary of those who generalize about them. Machines aren't perfect, but they have their place in a solid workout regimen like mine.

Macronutrient: When you eat, nutrients come in three forms: protein, carbohydrates, and fat. Most foods, and nearly all meals, contain some combination. As a rule, I like my meals to combine all three, rather than being overloaded with one. Carbs become especially problematic without the companionship of protein or fat.

Metabolism: The number of calories your body burns on any given day.

Negative protein balance: Woe is you if you find yourself in this unfortunate state, where your workouts break down more protein than you're taking in through your diet. To add muscle, the goal is to achieve a positive protein balance.

Old school training: Ever seen black-and-white shots in muscle magazines of Arnold Schwarzenegger and friends pushing around huge weights in Gold's Gym circa 1982? You can almost feel the chalk dust on the page. That's old school. Those guys were as strong as oxen and had the hearts of lions. I would have fit right in with those cats.

Overtraining: Go to the gym every day for weeks on end, and you'll find yourself in a state of diminishing returns. In fact, more training might be doing more harm than good. Often, overtraining is actually under-recovering: not eating or sleeping enough to support your body's heightened energy output.

Plyometrics: Any exercise in which muscles are repeatedly and rapidly stretched and then contracted. Examples: pushups with a clap at the top of each rep, and jumping onto and off of a workout bench.

Power: The ability to move an object or your own body quickly.

Powerlifters: These strength athletes compete in the bench press, squat, and deadlift. Unlike in bodybuilding, body aesthetics count for nothing in powerlifting, so these guys are huge and beefy. The goal is to push as much weight as possible in each event or lift.

Pre-exhaustion: This comes from old school bodybuilders. It involves starting a chest workout, for example, with a fly movement (a small move), and then following that with a bench press (a big move). By reversing the traditional big-to-small progression and "pre-fatiguing" the pectorals with flies, those will now fail along with the smaller support muscles during the bench. Otherwise, the support muscles will give way before all the muscle fibers in the pecs have fired.

Repetition: Taking an exercise from start to finish. Lift a dumbbell up to your shoulder and then lower it back to where it started. You've just completed one "rep" of a dumbbell curl.

Resistance training: Exercising a muscle or muscles against some tangible opposing force, whether it's a free weight, a machine, or a cable linked to a stack of weight plates. In contrast, isometric exercises and yoga don't rely on any counterweight for their effectiveness.

Resting metabolic rate: The total number of calories needed each day to support the essential functions (heartbeats, breathing, etc.) of the body, even in the absence of activity or movement. Survival would demand that the body burn these calories even if some Lazy Bones were to lie in bed all day long.

Slow-twitch muscle fibers: These contract more slowly than fast-twitch fibers. Slow-twitchers carry the load in endurance events such as running and swimming.

Stabilizing muscles: Everyone talks about training chest, legs, back, and maybe five or six other major muscles, but the human body contains nearly 700 muscles—many of which assist those bigger, better known drivers during various exercises. One of the advantages of free weights versus machines is that they force those stabilizing muscles to help out, a need that many machines eliminate with pads and seats. One potential problem: When you play a sport, the support isn't there.

Starting position: This simply refers to the fixed, motionless position that marks the beginning of a rep. The starting and ending positions are usually one and the same. Be aware that reaching a starting position sometimes requires some movement—for example, lifting a barbell to your shoulders before overhead presses—that's not part of the actual repetition.

Strongmen: These strength athletes flip tractor tires, carry around boulders, hoist cars overhead—anything that tests their brute strength. I've never hosted it (at least not yet), but The World's Strongest Man Contest is the Super Bowl for these unique athletes.

Superset: "Super set" would mean a really, really awesome series of reps, but the one-word spelling refers to doing one exercise immediately after the next without resting in between moves, other than the time it takes to move from one apparatus to another. After completing one superset, rest briefly and then, boom, repeat. Supersetting allows more work to be completed in less time.

Tempo: My program provides detailed information on the tempo at which you should perform various exercises, an underrated aspect of tweaking the intensity of a workout. Selectively varying the rate at which you move weight makes the same load easier or harder to handle. Slower is harder than faster. Slower is also great for unleashing the hormones that help to build muscle and burn fat.

Testosterone: The hormone primarily responsible not only for making men look and act like men, but also for building muscle. That's why you ladies needn't worry about bulking up. You have plenty of estrogen but merely a fraction of the T we guys do.

Thermogenesis: The act of burning calories to digest food. This process is one reason eating smaller, more frequent meals burns more calories than the traditional three squares a day.

VO$_2$ max: The maximum amount of oxygen your body can take in. Often used as a barometer of cardiovascular fitness.

Acknowledgments

Books are seldom produced in a vacuum, but this was more of a team effort than most. Along with paying tribute to my mother, father, and sister for their undying love and support, I'd like to single out the following individuals for contributing to *Mario Lopez's Knockout Fitness*.

So thank you to . . .

Joan Allen for taking these beautiful photographs. Your artistry behind the lens is a sight to behold.

John Damon for the use of your terrific gym Active Fitness.

Joseph Dowdell, CSCS, for designing this unique program with me from scratch. You're like a symphony conductor with exercises.

Justin Fortune and Freddie Roach for showing me the ropes when it comes to the sweet science. You guys rock!

Nancy Hancock of Rodale Books for believing in this project and seeing it through from start to finish. Thank you for everything.

Jeff O'Connell of *Men's Health* magazine for helping me to translate the thoughts in my head into the words on these pages.

Jimmy Peña, CSCS, for being the best trainer a guy could have and an even better friend. The sky's the limit for you.

Lisa Perkins for your constant support. People say they see me everywhere... because I have a remarkable publicist like you.

Andrea Platzman, MS, RD, for helping to design some killer recipes. I never knew eating healthy could taste so amazing.

Chris Rhoads for his remarkable design chops. You made this book fun and accessible with your visual talents.

Mark Schulman for the way you took an idea off the drawing board and turned it into this book.

Karina Smirnoff for teaching me how to dance, literally and figuratively. You are never less than an amazing inspiration to me.

Peter C. Siegel, RH, for helping me to help readers understand the meaning of the mind-muscle connection.

Kimberly Snyder for combining prodigious flexibility with precocious wisdom. You are wise far beyond your years.

Jim Stoppani, PhD, for helping me explain how to fuel up a body for great workouts and a long life. Your knowledge is unparalleled.

Eric Weissler, Esq., for making sure the i's are always dotted and the t's always crossed. Thank you for your dedication.

And last, but certainly not least, thanks to Tom Aczel, Suliette Baez, Marc Gerald, Jennifer Giandomenico, Chris Mohr, Blanca Oliviery, Marina Padakis, Ana Palmiero, Marc Sirinsky, and Matt Tuthill for your unique contributions. We couldn't have done it without you!

Index

Underscored page references indicate boxed text and tables. Boldface references indicate photographs.

Cholesterol, 10, <u>211</u>
Circuit training, <u>167</u>
Class, fitness, <u>167</u>
Coffee, <u>4</u>
Consistency, 225–26
Cottage cheese
    Cottage Cheese and Fruit, 153
    in Phase I sample meal plans, 75, 76, 79
    in Phase II sample meal plans, 145, 146, 151
    in Phase III sample meal plans, 212, 214, 217, 219
Crabmeat, 215, 218, 219
Crunch, <u>59</u>

D

Dance
    steps
        chacha basic in place, 200–201, **200–201**
        kick ball in jive, 199, **199**
        mambo spot turns, 204, **204**
        rumba Cuban breaks, 203, **203**
        tango swivels, 202, **202**
        waltz box steps, 205, **205**
    workout, 196–205
Deadlift, 181, **181**
Diabetes, <u>17</u>, 69
Dieting, 73
Dinner. *See* Lunch and dinner recipes
Dog, as workout partner, 88
Downward dog (yoga pose), 128, **128**
Dumbbell alternating chest press, 38, **38**
Dumbbell lateral raise, 109, **109**
Dumbbell one-arm row, 172, **172**
Dumbbell Romanian deadlift, 106, **106**
Dumbbells
    benefits of use, 7–8
Dumbbell split squat, 23, **23**
Dumbbell squat, 103, **103**
Dumbbell step-up, 115, **115**
Dumbbell sumo squat, 36–37, **36–37**
Dumbbell swing, 173, **173**

E

Eggs
    cholesterol in, <u>211</u>
    in Phase I sample meal plans, 74, 76–78, 80, 81
    in Phase II sample meal plans, 145, 146, 148–51

    in Phase III sample meal plans, 212, 213, 215, 216, 218, 220
        Spanish Breakfast Scramble, 220
Elbows, locking, <u>98</u>
Exercises. *See specific exercises*
E-Z bar curl, 123, **123**

F

Fast food, 64–65
Fat, burned by
    dancing, 198
    interval training, 10
    weight training, 5, 100
Fat, dietary
    in Phase I, 71–73
    in Phase II, 139–40, 143–44
    in Phase III, 209–11
    role in diet, 68
    saturated, 68
    sources, 67, <u>69</u>
    trans fats, 67
Fat burners, 65
Fat-free food, <u>66</u>
Fiber, 69–70
Fish. *See also* Salmon; Tuna
    omega 3 fatty acids in, <u>66</u>
    tilapia, 79, 212
Fitness level, 1–2, 4, 11
5 and a halfs, 136
Flat-bench barbell press, 182, **182**
Flexibility workout, 126–33
Focus, maintaining, 91–93, 99
Food. *See also* Meal plans; *specific foods*
    dietary mistakes to avoid, <u>66</u>
    fast, 64–65
    journal, 71, <u>73</u>
    sauces to avoid, <u>210</u>
    shopping for, <u>66</u>
Food poisoning, avoiding, <u>141</u>
Form, 18–19, 93
Four-corners drill, raquetball exercise, 136
Frittata, vegetable, 80
Front squat, 189, **189**
Functional training, 5, 6, 9

G

Giant sets for shoulders, <u>198</u>
Grapefruit, 73, <u>166</u>
Grapes, <u>142</u>
Gum, sugarless, <u>8</u>
Gym membership, <u>159</u>

H

Ham
   in Phase I sample meal plans, 77, 78, 80, 81
   in Phase II sample meal plans, 146, 150
   in Phase III sample meal plans, 212, 216, 217, 219
Heart disease
   decrease risk with tea consumption, 68
   increase risk with
      diabetes, 69
      sleeplessness, 17
Heavy bag training, boxing, 52, **52–53**
Hip bridge, 26, **26**
Horizontal pullup, 113
Hunger, 64, 66, 68, 140
Hydrostatic weighing, 100–101

I

Immune system, depression from lack of sleep, 17
Incline bench dumbbell press, 116, **116**
Incline neutral-grip dumbbell press, 191, **191**
Incline prone dumbbell "Y," 175, **175**
Injuries, 93, 113, 135
Insulin, 63, 66, 67, 69, 140, 143
Integrationist, weight-training, 6, 9
Intensity, exercise, 99, 99, 100, 156
Intervals
   advantages, 10–11
   basketball workout, 134
   biking workout, 56, 59
   lying down after, 19
   sports-specificity, 11–12
   timing in workout, 19
   work and rest portions, 10
Isolationist, weight-training, 6, 7, 9

J

Jumping jack, 105, **105**

K

Kick ball in jive (dance step), 199, **199**
Kidney beans, 142

L

Lamb
   Grilled Ginger Lamb Chops, 220–21
Lateral power shuffle, raquetball exercise, 136
Lecithin, 141
Lunch and dinner recipes
   Blackened Tuna Steaks, 153
   Dijon-Glazed Chicken, 221
   Grilled Ginger Lamb Chops, 220–21
   Oriental Beef and Vegetables, 82
   Salmon with Curry Sauce, 152
   Turkey Burgers, 83
Lying down, after intervals, 19
Lying dumbbell triceps extension, 110, **110**
Lying leg curl, 39, **39**

M

Machines, exercise, 7, 9, 10, 98, 100
Mambo spot turns (dance step), 204, **204**
Meal plans
   adjusting, 73
   Phase I, 74–83
   Phase II, 145–53
   Phase III, 212–21
Meals
   cheat, 140–43
   composition of, 67
   skipping, 66
   timing of, 64
Medicine ball chest toss, 192, **192**
Medicine ball overhead throw, 194, **194**
Metabolic disturbance, with interval training, 10
Metabolism, 62, 62–64, 140–41, 215
Mini-trampoline jogging, 111, **111**
Mistakes, training, 98
Mitt drill, boxing, 48, **48–49**
Motivation, 87, 88, 223
Mountain climber, 120, **120–21**
Muscle(s)
   breakdown of, 63
   fast-twitch fibers, 99, 166
   as metabolically active tissue, 64
   pre-exhausting, 167
   stretching, 21
   symmetry, 3, 5, 6
   weak, working on, 167
Muscle growth, 63, 71
Mushrooms, 142
Myostatic stretch reflex, 44

N

Nap, 224
Negative portion of movement, 98, 167
Nutrition. *See also* Carbohydrates; Fat, dietary; Protein
    fiber, 69–70
    metabolism, 62, 62–64, 140–41
    for non-workout days, 71–72, 143, 210
    for workout days, 72–73, 144, 211
Nutritionist, 159

O

Oatmeal
    Oatmeal with Stewed Fruit, 152
Obesity, 61, 159
Omega 3 fatty acids, 66
Omelets, 77, 81, 148, 150, 218
One-arm dumbbell row, 20
Onions, 142
Overtraining, 44, 98, 113, 135

P

Partner, workout, 88, 167
Pasta, 77, 81
Peanut butter
    Peanut Butter & Jelly Sandwich, 221
    in Phase I sample meal plans, 75, 77, 79
    in Phase II sample meal plans, 145, 147–51
    in Phase III sample meal plans, 215–17
Pecans, 142
Plateau, 113
Plyometrics, 44–45, 99, 166
Posture, improvement with dance, 197
Power, improving, 166
Pressdown, 176, **176**
Protein
    inadequate intake, 66
    for muscle growth, 63, 139
    negative balance, 63
    in Phase I, 71–73
    in Phase II, 139–40, 143–44
    in Phase III, 209–11
    sources, 64
Protein shake, 74, 144
Pulldown, 28, **28**
Pullup (assisted), 27, **27**
Pumpkin seeds, 78
Push press, with squat, 170, **170–71**
Pushup, 24–25, **24–25**

R

Range of motion, with dumbbells, 8
Raquetball workout, 136–37
Repetitions, 17–18, 98
Rest
    active, 10
    in interval training, 10
    nap, 224
    between sets, 92–93
    sleep, 17, 113, 225
Resting metabolic rate, 62, 215
Reverse crunch, 32, **32**
Reverse fly, 41, **41**
Reverse suicides, 136
Rice, 80
Role models, author's, 159, 161
Rumba Cuban breaks (dance step), 203, **203**
Running workout, 56, **57**
Russian twist, 187, **187**

S

Salad
    chicken, 81, 146
    Cobb, 76
    healthy additions to, 142
    taco, 146
Salmon
    adding to salads, 142
    in Phase I sample meal plans, 76
    in Phase II sample meal plans, 145
    in Phase III sample meal plans, 217
    Salmon with Curry Sauce, 152
Sauces, avoiding, 210
Seated cable row, 40, **40**
Seated dumbbell curl/shoulder press, 30–31, **30–31**
Seated forward bend (yoga pose), 130, **130**
Seated forward fold with bent leg (yoga pose), 130, **130**
Seated rope-handle cable row, 119, **119**
Seated spinal twist (yoga pose), 131, **131**
Seated Zottman curl, 177, **177**
Sets, 16–17, 98
Shadow boxing drills, 50, **50–51**
Shoulder press, with seated dumbbell curl, 30–31, **30–31**
Shoulders, giant sets for, 198
Shrimp, 80, 147, 149, 151, 213
Sidewinders, 136
Skipping rope, 117, **117**